Sex Without Tears

Sex
Without
Tears

by

Boyd Cooper, M.D.

Charles Publishing

Published in the United States by
Charles Publishing Company, Inc.,
Los Angeles, California,
and simultaneously in Canada by
Copp-Clark, Toronto, Ontario

ISBN: 0-912 880-00-7

Library of Congress Catalog Card Number: 78-190691

Manufactured in the United States of America

First Edition

To all the women who have played so
important a part in my life:
my mother, my wife, my daughter and
my patients

Contents

... Life demands that the duality in men and women be freed to function, released from hate or guilt. ... We need each others' qualities if we are ever to understand each other in love and life. The beautiful difference of our biological selves will not diminish through this mutual fusion. It should indeed flower, expand; blow the mind as well as the flesh. ... We could both breathe free.

Marya Mannes, *Out of My Time*

You can't hunt an elephant with a baby on your shoulder.

Margaret Mead, to reporters at the annual meeting of the American Association for the Advancement of Science, 1971

Sex Without Tears

A Personal
Point of View

Should a doctor concern himself exclusively with the medical aspects of a case and leave the moral and social implications to others?

This question was posed recently by a colleague making an address urging physicians to attend to their medicine and to restrict their attentions to the health of their patients.

As he concluded, the speaker received enthusiastic applause, in which I did not join. I could not applaud his views because I am in complete disagreement with them and attribute much of the public's increasing lack of confidence in our profession to just such narrow, shortsighted attitudes as this, among others.

I am an obstetrician and gynecologist, as was the colleague who made the address. An important, though not

13

usually considered, factor of my specialty is that my patients are all female. They come to see me because of sex-related problems, which range from contraception to childbirth, from venereal disease to menstruation, from abortion to adoption. Not one of these problems can possibly be isolated from its cause and its aftermath; in my opinion, every medical problem is a social problem and all too many are also economic problems.

As I write this, a woman of twenty-three in a southern state stands convicted under an 1868 law and faces a possible twenty years in prison because she chose to have an abortion. "I had rheumatic fever when I was nineteen and my mother died from it," she testified. But she can be given the same maximum penalty as someone convicted of manslaughter. How anyone, particularly a doctor, can feel that this woman's problem is separated from its social and legal implications astounds me. The operation was a success, but the patient may spend twenty years behind bars!

During the past half decade my personal and professional beliefs have changed drastically. The beliefs and attitudes of yesterday are gone; those which now govern me and my practice—and with which you will become acquainted in the following pages—are the result of dealing daily with things as they are, not as so many would like them to be or imagine them to be. I can be no part of the fantasy world which far too many people so blithely and blindly create out of the myths and traditions of the past, refusing to accept the social realities of the world in which we actually live.

The sex act can and should be one of the most joyful

14

and fulfilling expressions of the human spirit. No act, however, can be considered joyful and fulfilling when its aftermath may be tragic. Today, with modern pre-sex and post-sex techniques available to every woman—whatever her age, whether married or single—there should be no reason for the tears that all too often follow the sexual act.

I, of course, experience much more joy from delivering a happy, healthy, wanted child. Yet I firmly believe that an abortion can have aspects as positive as those of birth. Dedicated to the saving of lives, I have relieved almost 4,000 women of their fetuses, yet I do not consider myself an abortionist. I am sure that what I have done is right—it has been right for the mother, for society, and for the child who might have been. Mostly I have served the latter, for one of the most heart-rending tragedies of our age is the fetus grown into a child forced to accept a life of misery, rejected, neglected, subjected to the anger and resentment of a mother who never intended to have him and never wanted him.

Only the pregnant woman herself knows whether or not she wishes to give birth. The fetus and the mother comprise the closest, most personal relationship known to mankind. The decision, therefore, of whether or not to bring a child into our world is a decision the pregnant woman alone should make. It involves her body, her future and her life. It is not the rightful concern of government or church or her neighbors, or even of the father of the child, to attempt to decide for her or to influence her. It should, I repeat, be her choice and hers alone.

Sex Without Tears is not exclusively about abortion,

15

though that controversial, frustrating subject is completely and factually covered. I was motivated to write this book because I believe that we are beyond being at the brink of a sexual revolution and that today's woman, more aware and more demanding of her personal rights, is entitled to know all the facts relevant to her well-being both as a person and as a potential parent.

Boyd Cooper, M.D.
January 1972

I

The Quality
of Human Life

Times are changing—for women and for their doctors.

I have been practicing my specialty of obstetrics and gynecology for fifteen years, and they have been years of astounding change, not only within the boundaries of my professional world, but also in our entire society. It is difficult to believe that any other fifteen-year period in our history has made such a profound difference to women: in their opportunities, their expectations, and their perceptions of their roles sexually, socially, emotionally, and interpersonally. Old problems have been solved and many problems have surfaced. Though many old attitudes have stubbornly persisted, new ways of living also have been adopted.

Let me recall for you what it was like in a practice such as mine in the mid-1950s so that we can take a measure of what has happened to and for women.

The contraceptive pill had just been introduced, and it had seemed that the possibility of complete protection from unwanted pregnancy had arrived. The pill in its early form was crude compared to the refined variations that have since been developed. About a third of the women who took the early pill were miserable with side effects— they vomited violently and incessantly—but no one was worried about whether it might cause cancer or thrombophlebitis or any other complication. Today's patients, casually accustomed to the availability of the pill, are more sophisticated about its possible side effects but have accepted the statistical hazards as being within the norm for all medication.

Fifteen years ago sex among single girls was for the most part a closely guarded secret, kept even from their doctors. An unmarried woman who came to me for a pelvic examination was mortified to have me know that she was not a virgin, and if she arrived suspecting that she was pregnant, it took long and delicate questioning on my part before she'd admit to having missed a menstrual period. Today such a woman simply walks in and asks for a pregnancy test.

Most illegitimate babies then were delivered, not aborted, and most of those delivered were placed for adoption. There was no acceptance of the concept that a young unmarried woman might keep her baby. Today, though that situation is still difficult, many single mothers are trying to cope with it.

Fifteen years ago homes for unwed mothers were overcrowded. In the course of the intervening years I have seen these homes changing from punitive institutions, primarily offering concealment, to more open settings in which social-service casework and counseling are offered. This change is not universal, but it is becoming more and more widespread. In addition, today many of these maternity homes are closing up for lack of clients. In the old days pregnant teen-agers were kept out of sight and sent either to such homes or to distant relatives until after their babies were born. Today, instead of being cut off from school, parents and friends, they often live at home all the way through their pregnancies; in some cities, special public-school classes have even been established for them.

It was a disgrace fifteen years ago for a newly married woman to have a baby too soon. "The infant was premature" was the usual explanation behind which mother and her family hid. More than once I relented to anguished pleading and entered a low birth weight in the records for a bouncing full-term baby. Today some brides openly arrive at their weddings with protruding abdomens.

Fifteen years ago drug usage was not a problem, or at least not a widespread problem. Considerable usage was reported in the ghettos, which we then called the slums, but middle-class youngsters generally had neither the opportunity nor the impulse to dabble in drugs. Today we are so perplexed and tortured by the emergence of the drug culture that I find it necessary to ascertain whether a mother-to-be is addicted to drugs in order to prescribe proper procedures for pregnancy care.

These past fifteen years have wrought dramatic changes in me, both personally and professionally, as well as in my patients. Not only have my methods of treatment changed as new technology and medical findings have occurred, but also I have evolved a new personal philosophy that is utterly foreign to the attitudes I held when I first started my medical career.

As I think back, it seems to me that my present attitudes began formulating ten years ago, when I performed my first abortion, an experience I will never forget. My decision to do so was not suddenly or easily reached. I am a Mormon, and I had always approached medicine deeply influenced by the tenets of my church and the powerful traditions of the conservative medical profession. "Abortion," I assure you, was a completely negative term to me.

Though I had been specializing in gynecology, I had never before ended a pregnancy; nor had I given much time to theorizing or philosophizing. My energies had been devoted to building my practice and concentrating on the day-to-day problems that usually consume all the time of a young physician. Then one day in 1961 I received a patient whose life I would save . . . and who would significantly change my life.

Lisa was a vibrant twenty-two-year-old from Israel. Lisa was very much in love with her young man, and somewhere in their future were plans for marriage, but Lisa's problem at that moment was that she was pregnant.

For this woman, pregnancy was more than an inconvenience. It was a sentence of death. Lisa had heart disease as the result of a childhood illness, and she could not have survived a pregnancy, or delivered a live child. By the time she came to me, in her fourth month of pregnancy, the physical strain had already affected her defective heart. The cardiologists whom I called in for consultation agreed that she would probably not live another month unless the pregnancy was ended. However, four months is too far along for the routine type of abortion, which, under the proper conditions, is quite a simple procedure.

At that time in California, where I practice, a doctor could perform a legal abortion in a reputable hospital only if the life of the mother was in danger and if that danger was agreed upon by a committee of doctors. Today, despite a subsequent change in the law relative to the mother's danger, a committee of doctors still must reach an agreement. In Lisa's case the hospital committee, which in those days did not approve more than two or three abortions a year, had no choice but to agree that her life was in danger, and I was granted permission to perform the necessary operation.

The procedure, which called for an incision in the lower abdominal wall, was similar to the operation by which Caesarean deliveries are made, and rather matter-of-factly I prepared for surgery. I had done many Caesareans before and had the confidence born of successful experience. Then as I slipped my gloved hand into Lisa's uterus and cupped it around the unborn fetus everything changed. I brought the baby, encased in its sac, out of Lisa's unconscious body, and as I looked at it I trembled and broke into a cold sweat. Had this been a routine abortion early in pregnancy, I would have had little more than an unformed mass to remove. But, after four months of prenatal development, this was a perfectly formed miniature baby, with its legs, arms and head all recognizable. And, within its glistening sac, it struggled to stay alive. By separating it from its mother, I ended its life.

For weeks I was haunted by the memory of the struggling life that I had ended. What I had done was contrary to everything I had been taught in my home, my church and my professional training. The ethics of my profession were strongly imprinted on me, and they still are. After months of soul-searching, however, I found a new meaning in those ethics. I learned that the value of life itself, as a mere body count, is not the ultimate judgment for a doctor. I came to believe that it is the quality of life, not its mere existence, that matters.

I put an end to a life—technically, yes. But that life could not have survived. What's more, Lisa could not have survived. It had not been merely a trade-off of one life for another. Eventually I made peace with myself in terms of the living.

Finally I also asked myself some questions. Why shouldn't every woman have the choice I was able to give to Lisa? Why must the life of any woman be on the line before a pregnancy can be terminated? I recalled my experiences while I was on the staff of a home for unwed mothers. I remembered the feeling of shame and bewilderment of the girls trapped in a situation with which they could not cope; the times when girls were brought into the hospital emergency room after crude attempts to abort

22

themselves, bleeding so profusely that we could not save them; my shock in examining a girl disastrously infected and in severe emotional distress after she'd had an illegal abortion by someone untrained and unscrupulous.

What happened to the teen-age girl pressured by her parents to get married because she was pregnant, even though she was still too young emotionally and socially to understand what to expect of marriage? What became of the unwed mother who was told she had no choice but to place her child for adoption and who, even though she later married and had children, was torn by longing for the child she gave up? And how could you help the young wife who entered into the same sexual freedom her husband had considered his privilege for years only to find her marriage, her family and her future in jeopardy because of pregnancy?

In those early years, following Lisa, there was appallingly little I could do. I could not act outside the law, of course. But I could examine any woman who came to me suspecting that she was pregnant. And when a pregnancy was confirmed I could and did encourage abortions for those who really did not want a baby. And, most important of all perhaps, I could and did examine patients after abortions and render follow-up treatment.

Though I could not legally refer any of these patients to a doctor for an abortion, I soon developed a network of women who had gone for that purpose to Mexico, where competent and reliable men were available. An ever-increasing number of my patients who had been across the

23

border willingly shared the names of their abortion doctors with the newer patients. This arrangement short-circuited years of grief for these women.

The Pious Hypocrisy

Today, in California and New York and a number of other states, it is relatively easy for many women to get legal abortions. I unhesitatingly state that I do many myself. But the battle is far from won.

The law moves slowly. The attitudes of most people change at an even slower rate. Each woman is forced, therefore, to make her decision not only in terms of what the law permits but also in terms of what people will say. It is no secret that the deeply rooted prejudice against abortion still pervades this country. A simple and safe procedure that could alter the future of many young people is still viewed as sinful, a stigma, something to be kept as a shameful secret.

It is this barrier of mistaken beliefs and warped values that I want cracked. I am not primarily concerned with the legal aspects of abortion. Legalized abortion is slowly but surely being increasingly accepted throughout the country, and nothing will stop the continuance of that acceptance. What must change are the unspoken prejudices that seep through most people, the passing of moral judgments, the hypocrisy, and the costly and destructive cruelty that we piously inflict on others. I worry about the misinformation and misunderstandings that pass among Americans. Perhaps by sharing with others the troubled lives of some of my patients I may help to eliminate the overly rigid and punishing attitudes that still exist.

II

The Revolution —
Sexually Speaking

During the past fifteen years my profession has been overwhelmed by miracles, some of them so proclaimed by the sales forces of pharmaceutical companies, some by the press, and some by responsible doctors.

One of the most dramatic break-throughs, of course, was the authorization for widespread use of the contraceptive pill. Also introduced was the almost equally reliable mechanical tool, the IUD, or intrauterine device, which is inserted in the uterus by the doctor.

For many women, this turn of events indeed meant liberation—from fear, anxiety and sexual inhibition. Certainly today's new life style, in which sexual permissiveness is for the first time openly engaged in by many young women, can be dated from the advent of the pill, which has offered women a more decisive choice than ever before on the crucial question of whether or not to have a child.

The revolution has also brought liberation to women who still wind up unwillingly pregnant, although they are not always aware of their options.

What Are the Options?

There is no single wise decision for the thousands of women who still face the problem of an unplanned or unconventional pregnancy. Among the alternatives open to each woman are these: she can offer her child for adoption; she can keep her child and rear it herself; she can marry the child's father, usually under pressure from her family; or she can end her pregnancy by an abortion, which can be either a legal or illegal procedure.

Each of these solutions has its drawbacks and its hazards. No one is ideal for all. Each woman, as she makes her choice, should be aware of its possible physical, emotional and social consequences.

Pregnancy Persists Despite Contraceptives

There are apparently no simple solutions to the problems of a society in which legal, moral and economic issues compound situations that should be essentially personal and in which personal situations are themselves complex mixtures of physical and emotional drives and social and psychological pressures. And so, although we hoped that the development and widespread distribution of contraceptives to women would mark the end of unwanted pregnancies, we are far from that millennium. The truth is that doctors today are seeing more women who are unwillingly pregnant than ever before.

26

It's not that the pill has failed. It's not that the IUD doesn't work. It's just that the entire matter of permitting or preventing pregnancy remains shrouded in ignorance, fear, guilt and murky half-truths.

Most women of childbearing age do use some form of contraception, and for most of them the chosen method is effective. But there are still problems in selecting the right form of contraception for each individual.

Generally speaking, I think that the pill is the most effective and safest method of controlling conception available today. I rank the IUD as a close second. But in recommending methods of contraception, as in giving advice and treatment for anything, I am always mindful of the enormous physical, temperamental and situational differences among patients. There are some women to whom I make recommendations other than the pill and IUD. These range from the time-honored but now almost discarded use of a condom by the man to the newer and still not totally accepted procedures of surgical sterilization. There are also some patients to whom I have stopped making any recommendations whatever. These individuals are going to become pregnant—and remorseful or resentful or surprised—at regular intervals, no matter how much I advise them or exhort them or explain to them. They are simply pregnancy-prone, the same as some people are accident-prone. We'll talk about them later.

What We Know about the Pill

Compared with any contraceptive method we've had before, the pill is incredibly simple and convenient. It asks

27

very little of the patient: all she has to do is take one a day for twenty-one days, stop for a few days, have her menstrual period, and then start taking pills again. Nevertheless, there are some women who insist that they can't tolerate the pill and others who have been frightened into near panic by stories of dangers associated with it.

The pill is a dangerous drug only in the sense that almost any medication is dangerous, including even the commonplace aspirin. Any medication powerful enough to help you is also powerful enough, potentially, to harm you—that is, some of you, at some time, in some dosage.

The only complication definitely established related to using the pill is the risk that *some few* women will develop thrombophlebitis (blood clots). It does happen. It is, however, statistically a very low-grade risk. If those same few women had not taken the pill and had become pregnant, they'd have run a far greater danger of possibly developing any number of unforeseen complications of pregnancy. As for the other rumored dangers about the pill—becoming emotionally unhinged, becoming too fertile or permanently infertile, and developing liver disease or (most widely feared) cancer—there is as yet no convincing evidence for any of those claims.

It is highly discouraging to me that every time a medical scientist speculates in print as to a possible relationship between the pill and a disorder the report is widely publicized and hundreds of women lose faith in the pill. Journalistic indiscretion on occasion almost matches sexual indiscretion as a source of unwanted pregnancies.

There is little to fear, then, about taking the pill, though there can be a number of minor inconveniences: these are unpleasant side effects, ranging from skin changes and weight gain to nausea and break-through bleeding. Many times these side effects last merely for the first few months while the body becomes accustomed to the hormonal substances. However, it is sometimes necessary for the doctor to change the dosage until he finds one that the patient can better tolerate.

Who Should Use the IUD?

There are women who never achieve a comfortable adjustment to the pill. This group, of course, includes those who are phobic about all medication. There are also women who have valid professional reasons for not taking the pill. My practice includes many actresses and models whose camera-oriented lives cannot tolerate changes in skin pigmentation or even minor weight gains. For many of these women I consider the IUD the contraceptive of choice. It requires medical supervision at the time of insertion, but in most cases that's all the medical attention needed. However, I am not always eager to use the IUD on young girls, since they sometimes experience pain during the insertion; and I have reservations about its effectiveness on some older women who have had many children, because they tend to reject the coil spontaneously. Also, in a small percentage of women, there is the risk of infection or perforation from the IUD.

Spur-of-the-Moment Sex

In my judgment, the great advantage of both the pill and the IUD is that the use of either is not time-bound; that is, the woman is always prepared for sexual activity.

Since I am as interested in the emotional ramifications of sex, pregnancy, and their aftermath as in the solely anatomical or physiological aspects, this is an important consideration to me.

The diaphragm and all other contraceptive measures that must be inserted or applied just before intercourse have built-in temperamental hazards. The time or the place or the mood may not always be right, which can too easily lead to the classic case of taking a chance "just this once." Many women find the insertion of the diaphragm a distasteful procedure. Others insist that both they and their mates can feel its presence. Still others maintain that the spontaneity of sexual activity is destroyed by taking the time for the mechanics of contraception. "When you 'get ready' for sex the romance disappears," more than one patient told me.

Although, in my practice, I find very few candidates for the diaphragm, I think that for the woman with a very stable, predictable sex pattern the diaphragm is still a perfectly satisfactory means of contraception.

Teen-age Contraception

The young girl is a special situation. She is, in many instances, not liberated by the new sexual freedom but clobbered by it: she is catapulted into abundant and indiscriminate sexual activity before she is ready. She is also least likely to be protected by contraceptives.

"I didn't want my parents to know I was having sex, and couldn't hide anything around the house," one of the 17,800 teen-agers who underwent abortions in California during 1970 told me. (With 70,000 reported abortions, this means that over one-fourth involved teen-agers.)

Most doctors are somewhat reluctant to give the pill to a youngster who is still growing, since it can impair normal bone development. An IUD might give her some initial discomfort and perhaps cause some intermittent cramping. Despite these limitations, however, either the pill or the IUD could be the saver of life and sanity for many a teen-ager. These contraceptives, moreover, are available only from a doctor, and, unfortunately, far too few fourteen-year-olds are brought to physicians' offices for this preventive care.

At the high-school and junior-high-school levels sexual activity may be flaunted among one's peers, but it is not often shared with one's parents. And without parental sharing a girl is at a loss for medical advice and help. Such a youngster, the least able to cope with an unwanted pregnancy, is the most vulnerable. How does she manage?

A few girls, in the larger cities, may go to the free clinics where groups of progressive young doctors and nurses help teen-agers struggle with the problems of venereal infection, drug addiction and birth control. Much more often, however, these girls rely on the grapevine for "the best"— which usually means the least costly—way to avoid getting pregnant. That grapevine has come up with some imaginative solutions—two of which are the Saran Wrap condom and the Seven-up douche, neither being entirely useless. If I may make a contribution to the grapevine, I suggest that young men rely on the condom and that young women protect themselves with a sperm-killing vaginal foam. A

31

trip to the nearest drugstore for either product is all that's involved.

Is the Man in Charge?

The condom, I realize, has come to be regarded as ridiculously old-fashioned. Yet a case can be made for it. Its abandonment certainly is a major factor in the increase of venereal disease. Furthermore, within the context of birth control there are sound advantages, emotionally, to the use of the condom, despite its superficial disadvantages. Since the condom is a protective device, it permits the assumption of responsibility by the man, who can then shield his partner from the consequences of their sexual adventure. In fact, for some men, raised in certain traditions of maleness, it can be subtly castrating to be divested of this protective role.

Male responsibility is currently manifesting itself with an amazing increase in the number of requests for male sterilization. This can be accomplished by a relatively simple procedure—the cutting of the spermatic cords—which can be done in a doctor's office. The fact that it does *not* require hospitalization is an emphatic advantage, since most hospitals are still incredibly stuffy and difficult about all procedures relating to sterilization.

Will He Ever Be the Same?

When a patient tells me that her husband is considering having a vasectomy, I discuss the prospect with her primarily in terms of its being a mutual decision. First of all, I want them to be sure that they have really completed their family. Any vasectomy should be viewed as *final*. Although the procedure can sometimes be reversed, the patient must never count on it. The man must say farewell to future fatherhood, and he has to be sure that he is ready for that step.

There is no medical reason why the vasectomy, as a procedure, should affect either a man's sexual desires or his sexual prowess. But how it will affect him psychologically is unpredictable: in each case it depends on the total life experience and self-image of the individual. Certainly a psychological perception of himself as sexually maimed will diminish his sexual confidence. Fortunately, from my observations most of the men who choose to have a vasectomy appear to be very clearheaded about why they are doing it and seem to suffer little if any emotional damage.

There is, however, one aspect of the aftermath of the vasectomy that is often overlooked. Almost all men experience some dwindling of sexual drive as the years move on. Most candidates for vasectomies are men who have already had several children—that is, men who are probably in middle age. It is entirely normal, therefore, for a man at that point in life to begin to run out of steam sexually, with or without a vasectomy. As he becomes aware of this, he might tend to attribute it to his vasectomy, just as a woman who has had a spinal anesthesia during childbirth will use that as the cause for all future backaches.

A brand new type of vasectomy is presently undergoing massive trials in certain research centers. This method, if it proves successful, would permit temporary sterilization of the male. Thus he could in fact control the family planning.

The method involves the surgical insertion of a tiny plastic valve into the male tube that carries the sperm from the scrotum to the penis. The valve can be turned on and off by the doctor, thus interrupting fertility at will for any given period of time, short or lengthy.

The outcome of this method lies, of course, some distance in the future. That it possibly may prove to be medically feasible does not warrant that it will become popular.

If The Lady Is Willing

Surgical sterilization for women is a somewhat more elaborate procedure than it is for men. It means the removal of a portion of the Fallopian tubes, which are within the abdominal cavity. In other words, it calls for major surgery at about the same level of complexity as an appendectomy. If the procedure is carried out immediately after childbirth, it is usually more convenient, since the mother can recover from childbirth and surgery at the same time. But from a purely medical point of view it can be done at any time.

As is true of many situations related to pregnancy, there are roadblocks often placed in the path of a woman who chooses to be sterilized. In some communities there are legal restrictions; in others, hospital regulations make this an almost inaccessible solution. But it can be done, and in some cases it should be done. When is sterilization the answer? First of all, only when the patient is willing.

Second, only when she recognizes that no other way exists in which she can effectively put an end to childbearing. Such a case might be the woman who already has a number of illegitimate children, who is so immature or so unstable emotionally that she has never been able to use successfully any method of contraception, and whose tenuous emotional balance would be seriously threatened by the burden of more children. To her, sterilization would be genuine liberation.

New Methods in Sight

A number of new methods of contraception are being developed and tested. Among them, two seem particularly promising to me. Before discussing these, however, there is a relatively new method of female sterilization involving use of the peritoniscope finding favor with many doctors and at which we'll have a swift glance.

In this method, the peritoniscope is thrust through the abdominal wall, permitting the doctor to identify the Fallopian tubes. The tube is then severed with a tiny electric needle. The incision necessary for this operation is approximately one-half inch whereas, in usual sterilization surgery, the incision runs about an inch and a half.

The reduced size of the incision permits shorter hospitalization, a distinct advantage to the patient since it results in less cost and loss of time. Despite these plus factors, I do not use this method in my practice because I do not at this time evaluate it as being problem free. However, I will be watching reports from doctors who are using it in order to make a final evaluation for myself because it does represent a definite step forward in technique.

Let us now look at the two methods which are, in my opinion, particularly promising. One is, in effect, a "morning after" pill for the woman who, without protection, has been exposed to possible pregnancy. This pill has been available and known to be effective for a number of years, although it is not yet in widespread use. Its substance is estrogen, the same female hormone used as one of the ingredients in the standard contraceptive pill. When estrogen is given in large dosages during the first two or three days following unprotected sexual activity, it can prevent pregnancy. Perhaps it is more accurate to say that the morning-after pill interrupts pregnancy. To the best of our knowledge, the use of estrogen at this time interferes with the lodging of a fertilized egg in the lining of the uterus. Instead of remaining there and developing, the egg is expelled and the woman has a normal menstrual period. Not many physicians are as yet administering estrogen for this purpose, and not many women think in terms of post-sex rather than pre-sex protection. But the morning-after pill has great possibilities for extending protection to those who have been careless or forgetful. Its major limitation is that is works only if administered during the first two or three days following intercourse. Once the patient has missed her period, the pill won't help.

Perhaps even more noteworthy is a group of new hormones called prostaglandins. They are still in the developmental stage, but I predict that they will soon be available to all patients. For the first time, in the prostaglandins, we may have a safe and reliable manner of interrupting pregnancy, even when it is relatively advanced. An injection of this substance induces a spontaneous expulsion of the fetus in most women at any time prior to the time of normal birth. There is still a great deal about prostaglandins that remains unknown, but medical scientists are assiduously seeking all the answers. We need to know more about the proper dosages, the possible side effects and the after-effects. The substance's use on human subject, however, is already quite advanced. It seems to be entirely harmless, and eventually it may give us the most convenient way of terminating pregnancy ever known.

We can expect, then, that it will soon be possible, instead of using contraceptives, to rely on injections or pills taken after sexual activity. Today, with techniques of contraception developed to their present level, the means by which pregnancy can be avoided are many and varied, but it is nonetheless true that an end to unwanted preg-nancies is far from being achieved.

It is also true, as writer Gwen Gibson, among others, has pointed out that "there is no one typical, characteristic, stereotyped problem-pregnancy-prone female . . . they come from every socio-economic group . . . from the high school dropout to the Ph.D. holder. They come from the ranks of the married, single and divorced—and from the white, black, Asian and Mexican-American and the Protestant, Catholic, Jewish and Mormon communities—all in approxi-mately the same proportion that those ethnic and religious groups exist in the overall population."

Born of Laziness and Ignorance

The paradoxical situation of unabated high numbers of unwanted pregnancies despite the availability of progres-sive contraception techniques is indeed paradoxical, and to a certain extent correctable. However, I believe that overall the situation will continue to persist for as long as human nature remains as perverse and complicated and self-defeating as it seems to be.

Some girls get pregnant out of sheer ignorance. This is more likely to be true of the youngsters who venture into sex than of the more experienced women: some young girls are only dimly aware that pregnancy is a likely consequence of sex; many more are totally unaware of what measures are available to prevent pregnancy. If I were making this statement twenty-five years ago it would be received matter-of-factly. That it is still true today is outrageous.

For all the changes that have taken place in our science-oriented society and for all the lip service that is paid to the concept of sex education, ignorance remains a major blight. We have the know-how to present good sex-education programs, but the educators who have pioneered this effort have to struggle with the sanctimonious hypocrisy of many boards of education and self-styled community leaders. In many communities sex education is equated with immorality, subversion and the undermining of the home. How home and church and country are served by looking the other way while a thirteen-year-old child struggles with an unwanted pregnancy I fail to understand.

Ignorance is depressing but not hopeless. In my opinion there is less hope for the persistently pregnant women who seem to incur their condition out of sheer laziness. For some of these patients, what seems to be laziness is, of course, actually hopelessness. They won't make any effort because they have so little chance of improving their lives. I've seen them in the ghettos, where I spend a number of hours each week in community service. They are almost entirely unaffected by talk about improving the quality of life and not adding to the burdens of an overpopulated society. Since the quality of their lives has always been miserable, with society showing so little regard for *their* burdens, their reaction to pleas for birth control is a collective "don't bother me."

The Pregnancy-Prone Women

Another category of women indifferent to contraceptives is the group that might be identified as pregnancy-prone. Sometimes consciously, more often unconsciously, these women *seek* pregnancy, and I consider them the hard core of the problem of persistent pregnancy.

There is no single reason for pregnancy-proneness. The underlying causes are as varied as the women's individual life experiences. Let me simply suggest some of them.

The role of the little girl is a favored one in American life. She is cherished, pampered, adored and protected. It's not easy to surrender all that shelter and indulgence. It takes a bit of growing up. Some women postpone that painful step indefinitely, moving from Daddy to Hubby with very little role change. I have known women of sixty who still revert to baby talk and whose behavior is clearly that of persons who see themselves as adorable itty-bitty things. The woman stalled in her development at the little-girl stage never willingly gives up dolls, the enshrined symbols of her little-girl-ness. And for such a girl/woman, the sooner she gets pregnant and has a baby, the more assured she is of extending her role. It is no matter that there is no father for the child. Someone will provide. Someone always has.

Then there is the classic case in American life: the girl who uses pregnancy to entrap a man. She may use that strategy to get to the altar or to keep her husband from leaving her. A reluctant and entrapped husband might seem something less than an attractive partner, but apparently such a woman does not think so. Something in her past history has filled her with panic at the prospect of insecurity; her overriding concern, therefore, is to have a man in her life, for all time.

Another type of pregnancy-prone woman is narcissistically enthralled with herself. There are some women who actually feel physically and emotionally euphoric when they are pregnant, and these, of course, are not truly narcissistic; but the woman whose self-absorption leads her into pregnancy is. She is fascinated with everything that happens to her, and the drama of pregnancy is irresistible: the bodily changes that she can talk about with impunity, the early discomforts that mobilize everybody to her service, the sense of excitement and crisis as her time for delivery approaches, and the high drama of childbirth in which she is the unchallenged star. The narcissist revels in every minute of it and will go through it again and again. Invariably she makes a dreadful mother.

A girl's ties to her family also can cause her to be pregnancy-prone. Getting pregnant, particularly if she is young and unmarried, is a traditional manner of getting even with domineering parents or with parents who have lavished too much love on a sibling or who have belittled the girl and made her feel that they expect nothing but trouble from her. Sometimes, though, it's the other side of the coin that is seen in a pregnancy-prone woman: *because* she is tremendously attached to her family she gets pregnant. This is particularly true if her most profound emotional attachment is to her mother. She yearns to pattern herself after the mother she worships. What better way is there to do so than to enact the mother role herself?

There is also the girl who gets pregnant because her life is replete with a sense of guilt: having an illegitimate child will prove that she is really as bad as she suspects and the public humiliation will thus give her the punishment she constantly seeks. Additionally there is the girl whose entire experience with an unwed pregnancy is the acting out of a fantasy. Getting pregnant, in her dream world, is the expected consequence of making the scene sexually: it is the way to be grown up and to be part of the love world extolled by rock music. The major drawback to this fantasy is that it doesn't include raising a child. Thus the fantasy comes to an abrupt end with the reality of a demanding, needful newborn.

The Case of Lucinda: Pregnancy as Bargaining Power

Most of the pregnancy-prone women I see combine several of the traits I have sketched. For example, beautiful, redheaded, Texas-reared Lucinda used pregnancy not only to get her man but also to manipulate and punish him once she had him. Well on her way to a career in Hollywood, she became involved with Mac, a very successful man about town, older, wealthy and very resistant to marriage. Lucinda was determined not to go the usual route of her predecessors.

There was no question of her knowing how to avoid pregnancy: she was equipped with pills. But after a year of the affair she "happened" to forget to take them. It would seem that she had everything going for her: youth and health, beauty and talent, a budding career, and plenty of men willing to move in and replace Mac when he was ready to move on. But she was determined to have Mac for keeps.

The unmarriageable Mac, it turned out, didn't do battle, but he was most adroit at stalling. When the pregnancy was in the fifth month, Lucinda conceded defeat and went across the border to Mexico for an abortion. Considering the advanced stage of the pregnancy, she was risking her life; in fact, she almost lost it. She became my patient when she returned to Los Angeles and found herself bleeding profusely several days later.

A remorseful Mac married her when she eventually recovered, and I assumed that her case was closed. But two years later she came into my office. She was pregnant again and Mac was not the father of the child. She had been on location in Hawaii on a film and had had a brief interlude with a member of the crew. Hadn't she taken those pills I had prescribed for her? Oh, she had been carried away by tropical moonlight and the impulse of the moment. Clearly she was punishing Mac for the bad time he had given her before their marriage.

42

She told me that she would have the child and chance Mac's assuming it was his. But that blunted her plan for punishment, so she took enough friends into her confidence to make sure that eventually the news would reach him. The baby was born, and Mac has become very attached to it. Though he knows that the picture they present of a happy family is somewhat out of focus, he loves Lucinda. He believes that their problems are now behind them. However, considering Lucinda's view of pregnancy as bargaining power, I doubt it.

The Case of Karen: Pregnancy as Retaliation

Twenty-year-old Karen was equally pregnancy-prone, but for entirely different underlying reasons. A student at a nearby college, she came to my office to have her pregnancy confirmed. Examination advised me that she was almost in her fourth month and that it was not her first pregnancy.

With almost regal detachment she told me that she certainly was not going to marry the medical student who had fathered the child. She was well aware that her pregnancy was past the stage at which an abortion could safely be performed; she had quite pointedly bypassed the ready access to an abortion that the medical student could have provided.

In our first interview she seemed to lose her cool only when I remarked that she had been pregnant before. She told me with desperate intensity that she had placed her first baby for adoption and was determined to keep this one. In the subsequent months, as I saw Karen through prenatal care and delivery, the full story emerged.

The daughter of a faculty member in a small-town college, she had been raised in a home in which academic success and intellectual accomplishments were stressed and in which traditional moral and social values prevailed. From early childhood she was so acutely conscious of what she was expected to achieve that she felt that there were no areas of exploration open to her. By the time she was seventeen, she had decided to renounce the life of the mind for the life of the body. Hence she incurred her first pregnancy. It was her way of totally rejecting what she considered the stifling, rigid values of her family. Her intention had been to drop out of school when she had her baby. Instead, she had let her family take over, see her through her pregnancy, and arrange for the adoption. In return, she had agreed to go on to college, where, she assured me, she was overwhelmed with boredom.

Now she was again trying to break out of the family pattern, and this time she wasn't going to let her family arrange her life for her. She rather imagined herself as a modern-day pioneer woman, waging a battle at the frontiers of sexual freedom. In truth, she was a fairly classic rebellious youngster. There were, however, a few special quirks about her form of rebellion. For one thing, her feelings about her family were highly ambivalent. Though she scorned their values, she adored her father. Her devotion to him made it impossible for her to form a deep attachment for any other man. Both her lovers had been rather weak and passive men, and she spoke of both with contempt. Marriage, for her, was an unlikely prospect.

Another facet of her family history was the fact that she was very jealous of her two older sisters. Both of them

44

were conventionally married and rearing families, and she was determined not to follow their paths. In her mind, that action would be just another hand-me-down.

Karen had her baby and is raising it. She has left school and is supported in part by public assistance and in part by a small allowance that her family insists on sending to her. She is very much a loner, which seems to be her choice. I am not at all prepared to say that, with her temperament and her feelings about her childhood, she has made an unwise decision.

There is no correct decision for every girl experiencing an unconventional pregnancy. What is important is that each girl should have the opportunity to learn her options.

III

Adoption:
Pitfalls and
Plus-Factors

When should a young woman decide whether or not to offer her unwanted baby for adoption?

This decision should be made when she is the most rational and under the least amount of pressure. In my experience, the ideal time occurs in the second trimester—that is, the middle three months—of her pregnancy.

The first three months of an unwanted pregnancy are almost always a period of emotional and physical upheaval. Compounding the physical discomfort many women experience in early pregnancy are the psychological shock and the social pressures. First the woman has the uneasy suspicion that she is pregnant; then comes her reluctant acceptance of the fact that her suspicions are well founded, often followed by the painful experience of her rejection and abandonment by the man in the case. If she is a young girl, her family must be told, their disapproval and possible rejection must be absorbed, and the realities of "what people will say" must be met. All of this makes for a very turbulent three months, a difficult time for crucial decisions.

A Time for Decision

By the time the woman enters her second trimester, she is usually quite comfortable physically and has passed the point at which she can choose the alternative of abortion. She is undeniably going to have a baby, and usually the furore at home has subsided. She is prepared to face the future realistically. She should have the chance to talk out her decision calmly with her doctor and, it would be hoped, with her family and perhaps an attorney.

If she postpones her decision until the last three months of her pregnancy, it will be much more difficult to make it and to live with it. During that period she is very aware of the developing infant as a real, live baby and negotiating to dispose of it may be unthinkable to her. If a patient of mine has not reached her adoption decision before that time, I urge her to postpone it until after the baby's birth. Parting with the infant may prove very painful, it is true, but in many cases the harsh realities of taking care of the child by herself for many years are equally unwelcome.

We know the ideal time for the decision. But can we be equally confident about the ideal decision? That is a far more difficult choice. No two women react to the adoption experience similarly; the responses can range from great relief to inconsolable loss. Adoption does not obliterate the experience of childbearing, but time is a great healer. It is important for a woman to attempt to alleviate her traumatic situation by making a carefully considered decision.

The Case of Sue: Learning to Cope

Sue, when she first came to me as a twenty-year-old patient, seemed quite composed and in control. I would not have nominated her as a candidate for illegitimate pregnancy. She struck me as a young woman who managed everything very neatly. But that was not so. Her story was one of emotional chaos.

The daughter of unconventional parents—her father was a nudist and her mother was a lapsed Catholic who passed her sense of guilt on to her children—Sue decided to be a physical education teacher. Apparently stable, she was actually on an emotional merry-go-round. Her first affair was with a man for whom she was not ready either emotionally or sexually. Becoming involved with him meant accepting his persistent drinking and frequent interludes with other women. By the time she learned to enjoy him sexually, his constant humiliation of her was unendurable. The affair ended in fireworks.

The next man in Sue's life was rather low-key sexually, and she found it a relief. Then she ran into career problems. She was concluding her training and doing her practice teaching. Her future rode on the success of this practice, and she was under the supervision of a very hostile teacher. Sue was convinced that her prospects of obtaining a teaching position were going down the drain. During a period of despair she became involved with a new man, who was a notorious womanizer. Well aware of his reputation for carrying on with a number of women at the same time, she was also aware of having more fun in bed than ever before.

When she became pregnant, she knew that she had to face the situation alone. She cut herself off from her lover, her family and her career and left her home on the Eastern seaboard in favor of California where she became my patient.

Sue finally decided to give up her child. Following the baby's birth and subsequent adoption, she took courses at UCLA, got a job, and moved to an apartment of her own. She is now teaching in California.

Having an illegitimate child and arriving at the decision about adoption was right for Sue. She learned how to cope with life. To my knowledge, she has been doing so ever since.

The Case of Connie: Playing with Dolls

Generally speaking, it is much easier for young girls to give up their babies than it is for women in their twenties and thirties. Connie, a seventeen-year-old who lived in my home during her pregnancy, was ecstatic about the prospect of having a baby and hoped she could continue to live with my family for a year or two after its birth. She was one of the happiest patients I have ever known, and when she came back from the hospital with her tiny son she announced that she had everything she wanted in life. Some weeks later, however, Connie was going out on dates and appeared perturbed that my wife and I were unwilling to serve as baby sitters. Connie could not seem to understand that being the mother of a newborn was a round-the-clock responsibility.

When her son was two months old she asked me to arrange for his adoption. Having a baby wasn't quite the same, she had discovered, as having dolls that can be put capriciously aside, to be picked up when the mood strikes.

After the baby was placed, Connie moved out and found a job as a secretary. She is presently having the time of her life. Does she have regrets about the baby? Not at all. She made up her mind about adoption at the time that was apparently best suited for her, and she has had no afterthoughts.

Two Routes to Go

The adoption procedure is regulated by law and the details of these regulations vary from state to state. As a general rule, there are two courses to pursue: having the baby placed with adopting parents through a licensed adoption agency, and placing it by private arrangement between the mother and the adopting parents, with perhaps a lawyer acting as intermediary. There are strong points in favor of each method.

Asking an agency to handle the adoption is usually the preferred method for younger mothers. This arrangment is often made by the girl's parents, sometimes because the girl is totally unable to solve her problem herself, more often because the parents are overwhelmed by shame and want to be sure that all evidence of their daughter's "downfall" will be banished as soon as possible. It is customary, when an agency adoption has been scheduled, for the girl to spend the final two or three months of her pregnancy in a home for unwed mothers; also, sometimes the baby is delivered there. Expenses at the home are usually paid by the girl's parents but sometimes are covered by the boy's parents. In either case I feel that such payments serve as an expiation of a sense of failure on the part of the adults.

The agency adoption is part of the "system": it is professionally staffed, officially monitored, and built into our social service/legal/governmental structure. One of its strongest points, in my opinion, is that the girl is never aware of the adopting parents' identity. She officially relinquishes her child to the agency rather than to the new parents. This spares her, the new parents and the child from the melodramatic situation that can develop if the girl suffers post-adoption remorse.

Although the mother does not know the new parents, the adoption agency knows them in considerable detail. The agency spends a great deal of time investigating the would-be parents and does not place the infant in a home until it is convinced that the home is suitable. *Most* couples who seek to adopt a child are warm, compassionate human beings; but some, unfortunately, are warped and their motivations for wanting to raise someone else's child are unhealthy. Trained investigators are as a rule better equipped to identify these undesirable candidates for parenthood than are the young mother, her own parents, and even her doctor.

The Home for Unwed Mothers

In my opinion, the stable procedure of placing a child through an adoption agency would be infinitely more useful to many young mothers *if it did not require them to reside for a time in a home for unwed mothers.* I have had extensive experience with a variety of these institutions, and there is much about them that I have found to be negative.

Traditionally, these homes were established under religious auspices. Even today, many of them are more interested in saving the girl's soul and punishing her for her sins than in helping her to have a healthy baby and to develop a wholesome and positive attitude toward her future. The homes too often assume that the girl wishes to hide and that they are offering concealment. Many homes are staffed by well-trained, sensitive and perceptive persons, but many others are run by punitive, righteous and rigid personnel.

Some matrons manipulate the girl's situation by encouraging the father of the expected child to visit as often as possible. They are thus engaging in ill-advised or unwelcome matchmaking or attempting to inflict repentance on both young lovers. Matrons such as these are obviously not living in this century, let alone this decade.

The girls who live in maternity homes during the final, emotion-charged months of their pregnancies, isolated from all their normal ties, are also vulnerable to forming homosexual attachments. In some, a bitterness toward men lies close to the surface, feelings of rejection are raw and open, and a need to love and be loved leaves them highly susceptible.

From a professional point of view, I feel that girls living in these homes receive second-class medical care. Many of them have no prenatal care before coming to the home, and once there they are all seen primarily by interns or obstetrical residents from medical training centers. They also do not have continuity of care: often the doctor who attends them during delivery has never seen them before. Because of their youth, they are also considered high-risk patients who are much more likely to develop toxemia and other complications of pregnancy than are more mature women. Their physical and psychological needs require the most exacting and discerning professional care, which is far beyond the skills of most average doctors-in-training.

There are, on the other hand, some valid advantages to the maternity home. The youngster who lives there often feels, before her arrival, as if she has been sentenced to a term with a group of wayward girls, a feeling that results from our having categorized the illegitimately pregnant girl as a "fallen woman." However, at the home she finds not the promiscuous, wayward, "bad" girls she had anticipated but mostly girls just like herself. Sharing her crisis with others generally gives her, and her parents too, a new perspective, which is all to the good.

The maternity home also can often provide true shelter for the girl who might otherwise spend her pregnancy hounded by vindictive or reproachful parents. It is a helpful environment, too, for the economically underprivileged girl who would otherwise neglect considerations of proper diet and personal hygiene.

The Case of Jean: Better for Whom?

The best of plans made for a pregnant girl by her family, the maternity home and an adoption agency can backfire. I think particularly of Jean, the only daughter of rather young parents. Jean, a mature young lady of twenty-two, was no bewildered child when she became pregnant. She waited out her time in a maternity home. She and her parents were very close, and it was agreed that it would be best for all concerned if Jean's parents legally adopted her baby. They had always wanted another child, and this way they could have one. As he grew up, little Tommy came to understand that Jean was his real mother as well as his legal sister.

It was a happy arrangement until Jean married and eventually had five children of her own. Today she lives in a comfortable, large suburban home filled with lively youngsters. Tommy, now ten, longs to be part of that household. Although he is lonely in his own home, his grandparents refuse to give him up. He is permitted to visit Jean and her children often, but each departure from her home is a heartbreak. Jean is torn by both a longing for her firstborn and her guilt at having left him to her no-longer-young parents. There's no way for her to meet everyone's needs.

The Case of Tammy: What Went Wrong?

Tammy's story is quite different. When this fifteen-year-old child went into the maternity home I assumed that her child would be placed for adoption. But when she had her baby she couldn't bear to part with it. The agreement that she take it home to rear, with the help of her devoted parents, proved to be a disaster. Tammy has totally ignored her baby. Her parents, who were genuinely concerned with being helpful and supportive, find themselves with the full responsibility for the child. Tammy, with her first mistake so easily resolved, will almost certainly get pregnant again.

A Better Way

It is difficult to say who was at fault in the above two cases. Jean's and Tammy's parents both acted out of decent intentions. How can parents prepare to cope with the adjustments of a pregnant daughter? What seems to work best, in my experience, is keeping the girl in her own home. Adoption of her baby is often the best solution for such a youngster. She need not and should not be banished from her parental home. Her parents should say to her, in effect: "You are our daughter and we love you. This is our home, and we all live here together. You aren't the first unmarried girl to get pregnant; you don't have to spend the rest of your life atoning for it."

The daughter should be encouraged to be entirely open and honest about her pregnancy and her plans to have the baby adopted. She should continue to see her friends and to share in all family activities. Most important of all, she should continue to go to school, provided that the school system in her city allows her to. Many cities are now establishing special classes for pregnant pupils. If it isn't possible for her to go to school, she should be tutored at home. Dropping out of school during pregnancy can more seriously dislocate a young girl than can having an illegitimate baby.

Once the young mother has given birth to her child and the adoption agency has taken over, she should be allowed to continue to talk about her profound experience as freely as she chooses. She should not be hushed up or urged to sweep the incident under the carpet or told that the experience is over and should be forgotten. Above all, she should not be expected to behave exactly as she used to. She cannot be the little girl she once was. She may go back to her jeans and her sandals and her guitar, but she has changed and will never be the same again. She has become a young woman, has matured and ripened, and, hopefully, has been made wiser by her experience. She may be bored by some of her former friends, and some of them may shun her. She should be allowed to rise to her own level, propelled by her own new needs. Her parents should stay with her while the going is rough. After that, it's time to let go.

If She Seeks Privacy

The more mature woman, no longer a member of her parental home, usually resolves an illegitimate pregnancy in another way. If she decides on adoption, she usually prefers to do it through private channels. This method is just as legal as the agency adoption, and it has certain clear-cut advantages. For one thing, the adopting parents usually agree to pay for the expenses of the woman's pre-natal care and delivery. She goes to the doctor of her choice—or of theirs—and she has the advantage of first-class, private professional supervision. Because of a sustained relationship with one doctor, she can rely upon him for constant advice and counseling as she comes to terms emotionally with the decision to give up her child. If an attorney is involved in the arrangements, she also has his professional advice available. In short, she is more likely to act in a rational, well-considered manner than the youngster bustled off to an institution for unwed mothers.

Choosing Each Other

In many instances, in a private adoption, there is an opportunity for the natural mother and the adopting parents to meet in advance of the delivery and to take part in a process of mutual selection. Generally, such a mutual process is understandably difficult if the mother is a teen-ager.

The most charming demonstrations of a joint relation-ship between emotionally mature mothers and adopting parents were acted out in the home of my friend Hank, a successful young lawyer. Hank and his wife Barbara have an exceptionally happy marriage, marred only by their inability to have children of their own. About seven years ago I started placing illegitimate babies in their home through a lawyer, and now four happy children and two happy adults reside there.

The unusual aspect of this situation is that, prior to each adoption, the pregnant mother lived in Hank's and Bar-bara's home. Furthermore, after confinement each mother stayed in their home with her baby until she was fully recovered. Then she was on her own, with the unusual understanding that she was free to return to see her child whenever she wished, to watch it grow, to share it with Hank and Barbara.

It is particularly illuminating that, after the first year subsequent to childbirth, not one of the four mothers ever returned to see her child.

Some women who arrange for private adoption spend their pregnancies in the homes of others as baby sitters and helpers, as did the women who lived with Hank and Barbara and those who have lived with my wife and me. Most of them stay on the job until the day of delivery, and I have found this arrangement to be especially advantageous to the pregnant woman during her waiting period. Strain, economic and otherwise, is removed; she is busy, and in a home environment. She is therefore better prepared for the event of childbirth when she reaches the hospital.

It Is Always a Bereavement

Most mothers who give up their babies experience a profound loss, and almost all of them are left with a sense of grief. Nearly a year is spent in nurturing the fetus and birthing the child, and that experience cannot be forgotten. The intimate ties between mother and infant are not casually cut. There is, it is true, some feeling of loss in the experience of abortion too, but that is never as penetrating as the deprivation felt by a young mother whose living infant is taken from her to be placed in the waiting arms of another woman. Even teen-agers, for all their apparent indifference, are traumatized by this separation.

The emotional wounds of adoption after an unwanted pregnancy are, I have found, invariably cured by time. The human organism is marvelously adaptive. Most of us have an enormous capacity to adjust to the demands that life makes of us. Few young mothers who have gone through the illegitimate pregnancy and adoption experience are totally unscarred, but for most of them life goes on and, in many instances, even improves.

IV

Marriage for
the Wrong Reasons

Marriage is dynamite, more often than not ready to blow up.

Adolescence is a highly charged time of life, uneasy and unstable.

Pregnancy is a time of stress, even in the best of marriages.

Parental pressure on teen-agers converts normal rebelliousness into stubborn and resentful sullenness.

Combine these explosive factors in a forced marriage, and you have a bomb!

The shotgun marriage has for generations been the traditional way of "solving" the problem of unwanted pregnancy for young lovers. But it doesn't solve a thing. It almost never works out, and the newlyweds as well as the unwanted child are subject to lasting damage.

Doomed at the Start

Most forced marriages are doomed before they start. In fact, many of their hazards also threaten *all teen-age marriages*. Choosing a lifetime mate is, at best, a risky procedure; in truth, the choices made at any age turn out, ultimately, to be compromises. To expect youngsters to choose wisely is sheer foolishness.

Roadblocks exist in all marriages, since constant changes take place in both partners. Because of the inevitable personal changes, a man and his wife can become total strangers to each other in a span of ten years. If the marriage starts in adolescence, the alienation can take place in a year or two. Teen-agers scarcely know themselves, because they change from day to day, shifting in their physical and emotional patterns and in their personality structures. Therefore, with so little self-knowledge, how can they possibly choose their mates wisely? And once they make their choices, how can they know that the mates chosen will not, within a year, *in the course of normal adolescent development*, change into people they no longer know or want?

A really troubled individual in this dismal picture is a young bride already pregnant. Even a mature woman who chooses to be pregnant often finds that her self-image is gravely undermined during this period. Sometimes a woman cannot tolerate what she feels is the disfigurement of pregnancy; at times she even believes that her husband finds her repulsive and she becomes irrationally jealous and suspicious. A young bride, barely mature enough to manage herself, can rarely juggle the new relationship of marriage and the demands of a first pregnancy.

Is She Ready for Sex?

The idea that teen-age pregnancy is the flowering of an overwhelming love is, in my experience, little more than a romantic myth. Most youngsters are not ready for the complex experience of love. We make a great mistake if we believe that sexual permissiveness means sexual readiness. While many adolescent boys are sexually ready, the young girls brought to my office by their mothers are, although pregnant, far from sexually mature. Women mature sexually at individual rates. There are some who do not seem to be ready for full sexual response, physiologically or anatomically, let alone emotionally, until they are well into their mid-twenties. Others are distinctly ready at seventeen. The notion that most pregnant teen-agers are in the throes of the great loves of their lives is fallacious theorizing, not reality.

The Case of Sally: The Respectable Delinquent

Sally's mother had been a patient of mine for years. Sally was sixteen when her distraught mother brought her to my office to have a suspected pregnancy confirmed. Sally had barely started a sexual relationship with Paul, who was seventeen, and she was indeed pregnant. Both youngsters were from respectable, middle-class homes and were themselves thoroughly conventional young people.

Sally told me that because she was pregnant she guessed she was in love with Paul. There were some hurried parental meetings, and the two youngsters were married. They didn't particularly feel that they were being pushed into the marriage, and they didn't actively resist. It was expected of them, and they went along. Paul canceled his plans to attend college and went to work in his father's business. Sally dropped out of high school and, when the baby came, found it great fun to play at being grown up. It seemed to the two sets of parents and to the newlyweds as though everything was ending happily after all.

But Sally and Paul both did a great deal of growing and changing. Most of Paul's high-school friends went on to college, and he felt cheated. Sally, who had been quite immature sexually, had little interest in sexual activity with her husband. I put her on the pill, in order to prevent the fear of another pregnancy from interfering with her sexual responses, but that didn't seem to help. She confessed to me that she hated the idea of being stuck for life with the one man she had experienced sexually and that when she was in bed with Paul she kept wondering what it would be like with someone else. Paul, quite mature sexually, didn't wonder; he knew.

Less than a year after the baby was born the happy marriage was on the rocks. Sally's mother is now taking care of her grandchild as Sally tries frantically, and somewhat foolishly, to compensate for the years of fun that she feels she missed. She is finding out joylessly what it is like to have sex with a variety of young men. Paul talks about going to college, but he has lost almost two years and he fears that he has also lost the knack of studying. He is resentful of his parents and of the child whom he rarely sees. He could salvage all of his early hopes for himself, but he is in such a bind of bitter disappointment, of feeling that life is over for him before it ever started, that I doubt that he will.

The Hazards of Being a Child

The child of a teen-age marriage has very little chance for a normal life. Unwanted before birth, more often than not, he usually continues to be unwanted and neglected. Sometimes, however, he may be so indulged that he becomes excessively demanding and dependent. Either way he will have difficulties.

Social and environmental demands are not the only problems of young motherhood. There are also likely to be more than the usual physical problems. Statistically, women under the age of seventeen do not produce as high a percentage of healthy babies as the norm. The rate of prematurity is high, and a young mother may have to struggle with a very fragile baby. The rate of mental retardation is also higher, and young parents may find themselves trying to cope with an unending series of problems that would tax even the strongest of parents.

Further, if a young mother is underdeveloped anatomically, she may have an abnormally difficult childbirth and the infant may be injured as it emerges from a tight pelvis. Too often, also, such a mother's prenatal diet, normal for a teen-ager, is exactly what the doctor does *not* order for pregnant patients. Finally, the burdens of first-time motherhood are often complicated by a sickly baby.

Even when the baby is healthy, caring for it usually

deprives the mother—and often both parents—of the care-free, high-spirited recreation that is part of the normal life pattern of most young adults. In such an instance, the baby also becomes a victim of the deprivation. Often, because of the expense of baby sitters, the young couple will ask their childless friends to come over, thus making their home the base for their social life. Nominally, the parents are on the premises to watch out for the child; actually, the home often becomes a hectic, noisy shambles in which a miscellaneous assortment of teen-agers stays for hours or even, occasionally, days. Children do survive this sort of environment and, in some manner or other, "grow themselves up," but I am not prepared to say that they do so without incurring enduring damage.

The alternative to this catch-as-catch-can recreational life for the teen-age couple is to give up their friends and spend all their time at home. However, it is rare that both of them continue to remain at home. Usually the mother is left there, and that is the beginning of the end.

The Case of Irene: The Mother Who Disappeared

That is the way things ended for Irene, who at fifteen was happily involved in a romance with seventeen-year-old Dick, who lived in her neighborhood. Irene came from a Catholic home, Dick from a Jewish one. To their enlightened, urban parents, this did not constitute a barrier. The families liked each other, and by their mutual consent Irene and Dick were allowed the amount of freedom commonplace for young people today. By the time she was sixteen Irene was pregnant. To her parents, only one conclusion was acceptable: prompt marriage to Dick, the only boy she had ever dated in her life. Dick's parents were less enthusiastic about an interfaith marriage than they had been about an interfaith romance. They were disheartened at the prospect of Dick's not being able to fulfill his plans to become a physician. They crumbled, however, under the sense of righteous indignation that seemed to propel Irene's parents.

The young people, happy because they were in love, were married, and all too soon after the baby's birth Irene was pregnant again. Her religious commitment, which prevented her using contraceptives, also made it impossible for her to terminate the pregnancy. Dick, who had stayed in high school until he received his diploma, was then working at a service station and moonlighting on a second job to meet the expenses of his expanding household.

At her third pregnancy Irene became my patient. Then only twenty, she was a beautiful but discontented and restless young woman. By the time she had her third child most of the young love that had enlivened the adolescence of Irene and Dick was dead. Dick was working far too hard and was away from home far too much. Irene was bored with babies and overwhelmed by a diaper-festooned bathroom and a kitchen stacked high with dirty dishes. One day she simply disappeared.

Her parents, knowing that I had developed a good rapport with Irene, implored me to tell them where their daughter had gone. Dick phoned me beseechingly. But I hadn't the slightest idea of the young wife's whereabouts. I was as dismayed as they were, although not as surprised.

Some six months later Irene appeared in my office. She had taken advantage of her beauty and was being kept by an older man. She had renounced her religion, given up her three children, and cut herself off from her parents, and now she was rather wildly catching up on everything that she felt she had missed. She is currently living it up on the Palm Springs-Santa Anita-Las Vegas circuit, and she may well be the better for it. I am not sure. I am sure, however, that her three children are not better off for having been abandoned in childhood.

A Put-Down for the Father

Sometimes it's the man who, in the long run, is the victim of the hardships of an adolescent marriage. Few such marriages can be free of harsh financial demands and few young men are in a position, in terms of training or experience, to earn what they need. I have known some families in which the young mother could more easily find a job because of her readily marketable secretarial skills; the father, therefore, stayed home and cared for the baby. I don't think that there is anything wrong essentially in a father's bathing and changing and feeding a baby. Some fathers do those things very well and enjoy doing them, and that fact is not an assault on their masculinity. But, in our culture, it *is* emasculating for the man not to function as the head of the household. When a young mother is also the breadwinner, the young father's status is diminished; he will desperately need to regain his stature, even at the expense of the marriage.

Often, instead of letting the girl-bride get a job, one or

both sets of parents will contribute to the financial support of the young family. But that is not much better, in my opinion. That check from "home" tends to keep both young parents in the status of children just when they are struggling to make the transition into adulthood. The young woman resents her husband's inadequacy, and the young man is humiliated by a dependency he cannot shed.

Parental Hang-Ups

Many teen-age marriages are entered into willingly, but many more are forced by parental pressure. I have talked with any number of parents of teen-agers about this dilemma. Frequently when I talk with the mothers alone, I find that a high percentage of them are poorly adjusted both sexually and socially. Some parents who sentence their daughter to a life term in an unwanted marriage do so to punish her. These are frequently people who have never achieved a satisfactory sexual rapport with each other and have not been able to face up to that fact.

It seems implausible, in this day of readily available pornographic literature and "show-everything" movies, that Victorian sexual repression still exists, but I encounter it every day. I have patients who have lived through ten years of marriage in sexual reluctance and sometimes in sexual abhorrence. The wife in such a marriage is not likely to talk openly to her daughter about sex. She is also probably not going to give particular notice to the sexual burgeoning of her daughter in early adolescence or bring her into a doctor's office for contraceptive counseling. She will, in short, deny her daughter's sexuality as persistently as she denied her own. If she is faced with the undeniable evidence of pregnancy, she will renounce an abortion as a possible solution: she has gone through a miserable marriage, and that's exactly what she will impose on her daughter.

When both parents come to me, their hang-up is more likely to be social than sexual. In these cases, it's usually the father who does most of the talking. He is outraged; his position in the community is threatened. He is accustomed to managing people and things, and he is going to manage this "mess" in just the same way. His formula is to get people to do the "right thing" by his standards and then to move on to the next deal. His daughter also is forced into this mold.

The one thing that is almost always missing from these parental sessions is any input from the person most involved, the daughter herself. I am being asked to give her prenatal care, which should mean establishing an open and trusting relationship with her; yet her parents do everything possible to cast me in the role of their ally—in other words, the enemy. When I have the opportunity to talk with a girl alone *first*, I almost always learn that she does not want marriage. In such a case, fortified with that information, I am then willing to do battle with the parents.

Why It Doesn't Work

Do teen-age marriages ever work? The answer is less and less often in today's world. In more primitive societies, where the family unit is concerned primarily with survival, the chances are better. The young couple is so preoccupied with the necessities of food and shelter that there is little time or energy to examine their relationship and to question whether they are getting what they want out of life. The marriage partners need each other at the survival level, and they will need the children they are raising for the same reason: as more hands in the field and the kitchen. If the young people whose stories I have previously related in this chapter had had no other alternative, their forced marriages would not have seemed so stressful. If all of Irene's contemporaries had been raising families of three at age twenty she would not have become discontented. If a young man did not have to interrupt a promising career in order to manage a household, his drudgery would not seem oppressive. Today young people have many choices and many distractions. Survival needs are, in most cases, met at the push-button level; as a result, the rest of people's energies can be expended for purposes of self-knowledge and self-fulfillment. Marriage is no longer the only way to go.

Why Not Wait?

What do I advise for teen-agers who are pregnant? While many more of these youngsters are getting abortions than ever before, there are cases in which an abortion is neither advisable nor readily available. I do face many young people who are happy about their pregnancies and eager to get married and raise their babies. Even when a marriage is totally unforced, however, my advice to a girl is to wait. She should have the baby, by all means; and she should also have the best kind of environment possible during her pregnancy, even if that means staying at home with her parents. If a young couple is already sharing an apartment, that arrangement can often be continued. The ups and downs of pregnancy may strain the arrangement, but a marriage might prove to be a total disaster. Light house-keeping is easily dismantled; a marriage is not.

Following their child's birth, I ask a couple to come in and see me in order to take another look at their future. Ideally, this conference should occur a couple of months after delivery, when both young parents have had some experience with the presence of the child. By that time, I find many youngsters quite prepared to consider adoption; in fact, I sometimes find them willing to consider anything that will give them an uninterrupted night of sleep or a chance for uninterrupted love-making. But many young couples are absolutely blissful with parenthood and more determined than ever to marry, and for them marriage is unquestionably a good choice.

The Case of Mary Jane: She Waited

One of the most mature and well-balanced solutions to the problem of illegitimate pregnancy that I have ever seen was worked out by Mary Jane. She was twenty-eight when she became my patient and was certainly not the typical teen-ager trapped by pregnancy. California seems to be the mecca for out-of-state women who are pregnant, and it was Mary Jane's choice, as was the decision not to seek an abortion. She wanted to keep her child.

Did she want marriage? She wouldn't think of imposing it on the man who had been her lover. Although 2,000 miles separated them, they kept in touch during her pregnancy. He wanted to be with her, but she firmly refused. When she phoned from the hospital to tell him of the birth of their baby girl, he insisted, despite her staunch independence, on coming to Los Angeles to see her and the baby. He was eager for marriage. But Mary Jane wanted time.

When she left the hospital with her baby, the father found an apartment for her. After that, he went back home to wind up his affairs and then returned to share the apartment with Mary Jane and their child. Almost a year later, when Mary Jane was sure of herself, of the man's enduring feelings toward her, and of the capacity of both of them to be good parents, she consented to marriage. That was five years ago, and their marriage remains a happy one.

Maybe it's necessary to be nearly thirty in order to handle a challenging life experience with that much equilibrium. In any case, that solution strikes me as a very good one and I wish that more youngsters would choose it. I really think that they would, in fact, if their parents would just unload their psychological shotguns.

V

It's Not Enough
to Be Wanted

Not all pregnant single women want to give up their babies; nor do all of them want to get married. More women today than ever before *choose* to have babies out of wedlock, and even when her pregnancy is not a matter of choice, many a woman decides to keep her child and rear it, fatherless though it is.

From the mother's point of view this may be a very healthy resolution, at least emotionally if not always socially, but from the child's point of view it may leave a great deal to be desired. What we need, and do not yet have, is a solution that works well for both mother and child.

Who Keeps the Baby?

What kinds of unmarried mothers decide to keep and raise their babies? Those I have known run the gamut from wealth to poverty, from prestige to anonymity, and from the thoughtful to the irresponsible.

First there are the young mothers from the unconventional, "hippie" world. They seek to experience things naturally, including natural childbirth, which often occurs in their own lodgings with the father rather than a doctor in attendance. These girls are often adherents of health-food fads and participants in occult religious experiences and are almost always part of the drug world. They are seeking, often with the greatest of earnestness, a better way to experience life through love, and to them keeping a new baby is one manifestation of that love.

Then there are the young women who simply question the entire institution of marriage. They have sex partners with whom they may or may not share a household, and they want babies as part of their total experience. The pregnancies of these women are usually planned. These women tend to be fairly successful in their careers; some of them are even quite famous professionally. They are members of the establishment in terms of their professional lives, but they choose not to conform in terms of a formal marriage. They can usually afford to buy supervision and care of their children, but they cannot always afford the time and loving attention the children need.

A great many other young mothers who are rearing their fatherless children are welfare recipients; unfortunately, unless there is daring intervention on the part of society, the members of this large and growing group will probably rear another generation of welfare recipients.

Finally, there are the purposeless teen-agers who drift into sex, into pregnancy and into motherhood and then bring their new babies home to live with them and their parents.

Why?

A young woman from any one of these categories *could* be a very good mother and *could* rear a fine youngster. It all depends on her motivation. If the mother chooses to raise her own baby against social and often financial odds and makes the choice to care for and contribute to a new generation and share in that new generation's life, she has a good chance of making it. In other words, if she keeps the child for the *child's* sake, well and good. But if she keeps the child for *her own* sake, she's in trouble. So is the baby. It isn't enough for a child to be wanted: he must be wanted for the right reasons.

What usually motivates a woman to keep her child? One woman may do it because she depends on the child's love to heal her wounds of rejection by her lover, often by her parents, and sometimes by society. To such a mother her child is her most prized possession; she lavishes on it an intensity of love that all but smothers the child.

Another woman may keep her child because of strong prevailing cultural patterns. A typical case of this is when the decision is a young girl's parents' rather than her own. These parents, who have a strong sense of family, assert proudly that they will never give up their own flesh and blood. This attitude flourishes in many minority communities, where it is a way of closing ranks against what is considered a hostile establishment.

Keeping the child is also sometimes a desperate last-stand gesture on the part of the mother to maintain ties with the child's father. Perhaps she hopes that when he actually sees the infant he will relent and marry her. At the very least, she hopes, he will continue to keep in touch with her because of the child. Sometimes that strategy works, but more often it sends the father into frantic flight.

Keeping the child, particularly when brought into her parental home, can also be a girl's way of defying her parents: it is an eloquent gesture of adolescent rebellion. Sometimes the girl has a clear-cut intent to hurt and· to retaliate for real or imagined injuries; other times she has just a childish desire to "show them."

Having a child of her own and raising it is also the way in which a woman can reassure herself of her femininity. Many career mothers follow this path. Often this reaffirmation of femininity is a means of competing with a mother who has always dominated the family scene. It's a way of saying to the powerful parent: "What's so special about you, after all? I can have a child, too."

A younger mother's need to have a child of her own is often motivated by reasons of peer identification. What the others are doing she too will do. Nowhere is conformity *within the group* quite so relentless as it is among the young nonconformists, especially those of the "hippie" world. Many of these girls raise their babies in communes, which, despite their obvious disadvantages in terms of

75

standards of hygiene, at least assure the children of constant adult attention and enable the young mothers to share the burdens of child rearing.

Finally, many a young girl keeps and raises her fatherless baby because she has no other choice. Such a girl may be a welfare recipient or a member of a minority group living somewhat isolated from the larger community: she probably has been trapped from the beginning of her life, and motherhood is just one more trap.

No one of these reasons for keeping a child, no matter how much it meets the mother's needs, is a good reason, in terms of the well-being of the child. I have had patients living out each of the patterns I've sketched. More often, I have found several different motivations combined and intertwined in a single patient.

The Case of Rosarita: What Else Did She Have?

In the case of Rosarita, for example, it is difficult to know why she took the course she did. Was she compensating for rejection or was she one of the girls with no other choice?

Rosarita was raised in a bleak, dry valley south of Los Angeles, where she and her mother had been abandoned by her father, a discouraged migrant worker who returned to Mexico. The mother eventually found consolation in one of the many unusual religious cults that flourish in southern California, and in due course it became her turn to enjoy the sacred privilege of being the bed partner of the leader of the cult.

By the time she was a ripe twelve, Rosarita herself was

summoned by the leader to replace her mother. An outraged, distraught and, above all, wildly jealous mother
banished her daughter, and Rosarita took to the road,
headed for Los Angeles. The first man who picked up the
young hitchhiker took her to a hotel, and after that the
pattern of her life was pretty well set. She drifted from
man to man. At one point she was so emotionally assaulted by her sense of abandonment that she was committed to a state mental hospital. I first met her there,
during a gynecological research project in which I was
involved. To me the most wistful thing about Rosarita was
the fact that she felt safer and more at home in the hospital than in the outside world.

After her discharge she went to San Francisco, where
she found a home of sorts in the drug culture of Haight-
Ashbury. There she met Jake, a rock musician. "I found
love on acid," she later told me, "and I was happy doing
what Jake called 'the woman thing.' " She lost Jake when
he was arrested, but in the brief and rather happy interim
she had become pregnant. She kept her baby through a
sordid cycle of no money, no man and no home.

Back in Los Angeles, she tried to support her child by
baby-sitting, but eventually she went back to hustling.
When she became pregnant again she applied for public
assistance.

She came to see me for prenatal care, bringing along her
beautiful and treasured little son. I tried to talk with this
life-battered nineteen-year-old, hoping to work out a more
rational solution for her and her babies. But the idea of
giving them up—even for their own good—was not accept-

able to her. Rosarita offered stony, cold refusal, then tears. Clearly, both the baby she already had and the one on its way were everything to her. They were making up for the father who had deserted her, the mother who had renounced her, the "great love" who had copped out, and the scores of other men who were nameless and faceless.

Rosarita is now raising both her children in a makeshift, marginal manner. That is her answer to life.

The Case of Clare: No Longer in Judgment

Clare's reasons for having her child and raising it as an unmarried professional woman are quite different. So is Clare's life story.

The duaghter of a domineering father and a patient, put-upon mother, Clare decided early not to pattern herself after her mother. The demeaning role of a housewife was not for her. She decided to study law, and she did so, drivingly, almost at a level of self-punishment. That was, for Clare, a way to unshackle herself from the hated role of woman. At law school in the Pacific Northwest she met and married a young law clerk. Somehow, however, she hadn't given much thought to the sexual commitment of marriage, and she quite literally fought it. The wedding night engendered a brutal quarrel, and at four in the morning the bridegroom walked out. Clare, with considerable emotional support from her father, had the marriage annulled.

From that point on, Clare poured everything into her career. Eventually, still quite young, she became one of the few women judges in her state. Because of her professional prominence, she received a considerable amount of attention from the news media; ultimately she became close friends with Rick, a brilliant television newscaster. Rick was based in New York, but his assignments often brought him to the West Coast, where he was away from his wife and available to Clare. To Clare, the relationship was not a romance but just one of a series of stimulating friendships with challenging men; but that wasn't how Rick saw it. He romanced her in a fairly typical way: gifts, dinners, and parties with friends. Since Clare seemed to enjoy it all, Rick interpreted her feelings as encouragement. Eventually, he collected what he felt was his due; but in Clare's terms she was raped.

When she suspected that she was pregnant, Clare came to southern California and made an appointment with me. When I confirmed her pregnancy, her uppermost feeling was that "this awful thing couldn't be happening to me." How ironic, I thought, that someone who sat in judgment professionally could have so little understanding of either herself or the world in which she was functioning.

Three weeks later Clare announced to me that she had decided to have her child and to keep it. She had spent the intervening time virtually alone, in an apartment that she had rented for herself, reviewing her life. Most of that life, she felt, had been spent denying her femininity, and this child, she had finally concluded, might be her only chance to affirm it. She had enjoyed a range of experiences and satisfactions traditionally reserved for men, so why should she not also enjoy the one that is uniquely a woman's?

Clare resigned from her judgeship and moved to Los

Angeles, and she is now practicing corporate law with a large firm. Her little daughter lives with her, under the supervision of a housekeeper. Clare, still very busy and very much an operator in a man's world, doesn't have a great deal of time to spend with the child, but their hours together do seem joyous. Clare feels fulfilled, but about the child's feelings one can't be sure.

The Case of Kathy: One Big Happy Family

Kathy has kept her baby, too, though I feel that somehow she has been sidetracked from the actual experience of raising a child. The youngest of a large Irish Catholic family, Kathy was a bouncy, attractive adolescent. Like many youngsters with her background, she had daydreamed for a time about joining a religious order. That phase had passed, but she had remained a devoutly religious girl.

Her family was delighted when she started going steady with Tony, whose Italian Catholic family was as warm and loving as Kathy's. Kathy and Tony were part of a large, closely knit crowd, and most of their time together was spent in such exuberant group pleasures as surfing and skiing. It could not have been a more wholesome situation, nor one more certainly headed for a church wedding.

The courtship lasted for four years, with both young people ardent but held in check by both their own religious scruples and a fair degree of parental control. Eventually the familiar problem presented itself to Tony. Now a man, he could no longer postpone sexual gratification. For Kathy, however, waiting until after the wedding was no problem at all. Thus it happened that another girl, someone outside the crowd, entered the picture and readily offered Tony what Kathy had denied him.

When Kathy found out, she fought for her man in classic fashion. She decided to beat her rival on her terms. At a weekend excursion of the group she planned her strategy carefully and spent the night sharing a sleeping bag with Tony. After the episode was over, she was embarrassed, ill at ease and tearful, but she was also confident that, once and for all, she had sealed her future with Tony.

Tony, however, decided that sex was simpler, and actually more fun, with his other girl. And then Kathy discovered that she was pregnant. She was referred to me by a colleague, who had been her pediatrician.

Kathy arrived at my office with her mother, and it was clear that the family had closed ranks. Tony had disappeared, but Kathy's mother was undaunted. Of course her little girl would have her baby; in fact, she would keep both Kathy and the baby right there at the family hearth. "After all," she said, "there's always room for one more darling baby in a family as large as ours."

The child is now being raised mostly by Kathy's mother, a woman no longer young, in a home where there are no other children. Kathy is in and out, sometimes working at out-of-town jobs, sometimes living at home trying to make up for lost time with her baby. She feels isolated from the old crowd, is still very wounded at being discarded by Tony, and believes that she ought to find a husband so that she can make a home for her child. But the child's real ties seem to be with the grandmother; the family arranged it that way.

Solitary Child Rearing Is Rough

All three of these women chose to keep their babies. And, in one sense, it can be said that they made their decisions for the wrong reasons. They were responding to their own needs rather than to the needs of their children. In all fairness, however, I must concede this point: *no matter what her motivation*, the woman alone who tries to rear a child has a very rough time. This is true for any woman, whether she is single, divorced or widowed. We have, in American society, very little to offer such a woman in order to make her task easier. We behave as though the problem were hers alone and not ours at all.

As things now stand, the single mother has the cards stacked against her. She can rarely do a good job as a mother, and the obligation of being the breadwinner is usually too much of a burden. If she is able to get a job or enroll in a job-training program, she can give her child only fragmented mothering. In some instances, she can place her preschool child in a day-care center, where he receives limited and uneven attention. But once the child is old enough to go to public school he becomes a member of the desolate army of latchkey children, shifting for himself when school is out. Another choice for such a mother is to embark on the endless process of negotiating with a series of baby sitters and passing the child around from one adult to another, many of them unpredictable and unreliable, some of them even unstable.

If such a mother does not work, either because she has no skills or because she has no way of providing care for her baby, she will, more likely than not, become a welfare recipient and, automatically, an overworked target for public indignation. One is asked to believe that such a woman industriously produces one illegitimate child after another, just to boost the size of her relief check, and that her life is devoted to deceiving the authorities, particularly about the presence or absence of a man in her household. My experience convinces me—and I have provided professional care to many women on welfare—that most of these women *do not want* to go on welfare and definitely *do not want* to remain there. Such patients tell me that they find receiving welfare assistance a degrading and humiliating experience that is far from a financial windfall. Most of them long for an alternate way. In the next chapter I am going to suggest a solution that, I believe, merits extensive study—a possible solution, not only for women on relief, but for all single mothers.

VI

A Proposed
Solution for
the Single Mother

I propose that there be established in this country a network of *children's centers*. What I have in mind are *not* day-care centers. The existing institutions are, in many locations, doing a very good job, and many more of them will probably be opened in the next ten years. But these centers are designed primarily to care for only certain children—those of preschool age—and to serve only certain mothers—those who work.

The centers that I have in mind would serve a much wider range of children and mothers. They would be open not only during the workday but twenty-four hours a day, seven days a week, although no child would be expected to stay there all the time. They would provide more than day care by operating as centers for learning, growing and living—for both the children and the mothers. They would be publicly supported: while many women would pay for their services, those who could not pay would receive the services without charge.

Centers similar to the ones I have in mind are now operating in a number of European countries and elsewhere in the world. Many mistakes have been made in such programs, and many problems have been encountered. We can already benefit from such experiences and build an improved American model.

I am not proposing that we let the government take over the mother/child relationship; I am just suggesting that we ask the government to strengthen that relationship. I am not advocating an institution that supplants the home and family; I am proposing one that supplements it.

How It Would Work

Let's see how such a center would actually work. Let's take the case, for example, of an unmarried, pregnant, jobless, impoverished girl.

She would enroll in the center as soon as her pregnancy was determined; ideally, she would be referred there by her public-assistance caseworker. At the center her training as a mother would begin. She would learn the elements of sound prenatal health practices. She would share in group counseling with other young women, some in various stages of unmarried pregnancy, others who would already have given birth to their babies. The counseling would prepare her for her immediate future as an unmarried mother keeping her child. It would also help her explore the broader and deeper problems of who she is, how she characteristically deals with life situations, what she really wants out of life, and how changes in her behavior might bring her closer to her goals.

Her pregnancy would be lived in an open, honest, shame-free environment such as few young women now enjoy. Vocational counseling would help her develop realistic plans for the kind of work she might be trained to do after having her baby.

All through her pregnancy she would work at the center, caring for young children and learning how to do this skillfully. Many of these young women, I predict, would receive deep satisfaction from mothering children, and they could, if they chose to do so, stay on as part of the center staff after having their babies. Thus one of society's most sorely needed skills—that of expert child rearing—would no longer be supplied on a hit-or-miss basis but would be elevated to almost the level of a profession.

When a girl has had her baby, she would be able to keep it at the center while she prepared herself for economic independence. At the center the child would have an infinitely better environment than it could possibly have if the mother kept it at home with her all day. It would be well nourished and would share with other children the experience of developing and growing. The center, however, would *not* be a dumping ground for children. No child would stay there all day every day.

Typically, a young mother would spend part of each day with her own child, perhaps at the end of her work day; but that schedule would be flexible. Even the most conscientious and devoted young mother needs some time to herself, and this need is not limited to unmarried mothers. I have known many married mothers who get a great deal of child-rearing help from their husbands but who, nevertheless, are made frantic by the day-to-day demands of caring for their children. This desperation is immeasurably more acute for the young working mother with no husband to help her. If, after work, she wants to go out on a date or if she wants to spend a weekend with a man, she ought not to be perpetually frustrated by the fact that she has a child. The children's center should have some staff on hand all the time so that, on occasion, a child can be left there during evening hours or overnight.

The kind of freedom that a young mother would have when her child is at the center would benefit both the mother and the child. If the needs of the child do not become burdensome to the mother, if she can shape her life with some independence, the relationship between the mother and the child would be more likely to be loving and supportive. The time they would spend together in the mother's home would be not a resented imprisonment but an experience of joyful exploration of each other.

One of the gravest deprivations of the welfare child is the absence of models after whom he can pattern a decent life for himself. Strengthened by what she would learn in the center, the mother would become a better model. She would be less likely to resort to drink or drugs, slovenliness and chronic dependence. Most important of all, there would be men in the day-to-day environment at the center; they would be doctors, psychologists, counselors and recreation directors. Thus the fatherless child would not grow up bereft of a male model.

Not a Cure-All

I do not think that such a children's center would be the panacea of all our problems. Some children might be difficult to handle because they are emotionally disturbed and might be threatening to other children. There would also be the risk that some children would be brought in with infectious diseases and might endanger others. But these are problems that occur in any home and any neighborhood, and they could be dealt with better in a center with a medical staff to examine the children, a small inpatient ward for children who should be kept in bed, and psychological consultants to help stabilize those who are disturbed.

Less easily solved would be the need for a developing child to have a strong, *continuing* relationship with at least one adult through his childhood years. I would hope that the child's own mother could serve that role even though she would be away from the child for part of each day; and I am convinced that she would do a better job as a mother if she fulfilled the role through choice rather than through obligation.

The primary beneficiaries of the network of children's centers would be unmarried mothers living in economic distress, but I can anticipate many others as well. The young widow or divorcee with small children needs help too. Even though she may receive money for child support—in which case she can pay the center—her child may need daytime care while she works and occasional evening care while she goes out. A young widowed father is also frequently quite frantic for help, and often he makes a hasty and unwanted marriage primarily to get a home-maker. The center would help him too. In addition, many a happily married woman is more career-minded than home-minded and resents the fact that her talents and training are going to waste while she impatiently waits for her children to grow up. If such a woman could count on a center to provide good care for her children, she too would be a happier woman and a better mother.

It is likely that she would be a healthier woman as well. Perhaps it's no mere accident that the country in which a female can look forward to the greatest life expectancy in the world, Sweden, is also a country whose people are not uptight about sexual freedom, and which offers exactly the type of child care centers discussed in this chapter. (According to the latest issue of the United Nations Demographic Yearbook, Swedish girls have a life expectancy of 76.5 years. It might also be noted that the life expectancy of the Swedish male likewise leads the world, 71.9 years.)

An End to Illegitimacy

If the kind of children's center I have envisioned is going to work for the good of *all* children, if it is indeed going to be a means of breaking the welfare cycle, it will have to be accompanied by yet another bold change. This change is the abolishment of the concept of illegitimacy in our legal system. There must be no differentiation between a child born in wedlock and one born out of it. Here, again, I am suggesting that we open-mindedly examine the practices of countries that have already taken this step. All children, regardless of the circumstances of their births, should have the same rights and be entitled to the same protection.

The Case of Inga: This Country Failed Her

It came as quite a shock to one of my patients to find out how much this country differed from her own. Inga came from Sweden, lived and worked here, and felt very much at home. She still had ties to her old country, and she earned enough money so that she could go back there for a month's vacation every second year, but she had a more compelling tie here, a married man with whom she was very much in love. The man's marriage had burned itself out, but he was deeply involved with his four young children and for him divorce was out of the question. But Inga could easily settle for that: the affair gave her most of what she needed sexually and emotionally.

After being on the pill for five years, Inga panicked when she read an inflammatory article in a newspaper about the complications that may follow its use. She went off the pill, but she neglected to replace it with another contraceptive device. As a result, at age forty-two Inga became pregnant. She pondered her dilemma and decided that she might be experiencing her last chance at mother-hood. She also loved her man and wanted his child; but she did not anticipate how her total life style would change.

First she lost her job, because her boss had had disas-trous experiences with women employees who had small

90

children to care for: he had seen too many crises, too many days when an employee didn't show up. For someone working at Inga's level of responsibility, he said, this behavior wouldn't do. Jobless, Inga began to explore how women manage with fatherless children. What she found was very dismal indeed. She learned that all she could count on was a meager welfare check and the prospect of spending her time doing nothing but child rearing. But she knew that there was a better way, because she had seen it work in Sweden; and so she took her child and went back to her old country for the sort of decent, dignified shelter and opportunity that this country does not provide for its unmarried mothers.

We punish, in scores of demeaning, judgmental ways, single women who get pregnant. We punish both the mother and the child when a woman decides to keep her baby. In fact, only recently are we beginning to abate our punishment of a woman who is pregnant and *does not want to have a child*. Let's look now at the paths that can be traveled by a woman for whom the only solution is an abortion.

VII

The Self-Induced Abortion

It is not impossible for a girl to perform an abortion on herself. The chances are deplorably high, however, that she will not only destroy the fetus but end her own life as well. The subject of self-induced abortion should not be discussed casually. Such an abortion is the most dangerous way to terminate a pregnancy and usually produces serious physical and psychological consequences.

The techniques of self-induced abortion can be classified in three categories: insertion, ingestion and exertion. The first of these is potentially very hazardous and the other two are relatively harmless and utterly ineffective.

Ignorance Is Not Bliss

Why would a young woman embark on such a doomed course as self-induced abortion? Often the reason is pure ignorance. She learns that she is pregnant and doesn't know how to extricate herself from her plight. She may not know that a doctor can and usually will help her; in fact, if she is without money, public facilities for help are available. She may talk to friends about her problem and hear something that sounds like a sure-fire method and, in her troubled state, her ignorance may permit her to consider the suggestion because she *does not know* how dangerous the method might be.

Another young woman may react to her pregnancy as she customarily reacts to an illness, with self-diagnosis and self-treatment. It may be characteristic for her to think that she shouldn't bother the doctor with her problem and that she can take care of it herself. Whatever a woman's reason for self-abortion, part of it is ignorance. Fortunately, however, ignorance is a treatable disorder, so I sincerely hope that these pages will be therapeutic to those with misguided views.

Poverty is another reason often given to explain the crude and cruel methods by which women have attempted to terminate pregnancy. Often poverty and ignorance go hand in hand. An impoverished woman may fail to seek a doctor and an abortion because she fears that doing so may cause cancellation of public assistance. Actually, separate monies are available for a legal abortion through public funds. In fact, many caseworkers in welfare agencies will help their clients obtain such treatment.

The Self-Destructive Drive

Ignorance we can cope with. Poverty, to a large extent, we can also alleviate. The third type of woman likely to induce her own abortion is quite another problem—invariably a difficult case to reach. She is the psychologically disturbed person. The violence she does to herself in self-abortion all too neatly satisfies her unstable emotional needs. How many self-damaged women fall into this category cannot be estimated, since most of them do not come to a doctor for help either before or after the self-abortion. That's part of their problem. They will not seek help from anyone.

Typically highly withdrawn and introspective, such a woman usually has a strong drive toward self-destruction. Her personality structure includes a debased self-image. She got pregnant to demonstrate that she's no good, and she righteously punishes herself by getting rid of her fetus, no matter what the risks are. The masochism that is part of this syndrome goes to great lengths. I had one patient who had brutally beaten herself on the abdomen during the early weeks of her pregnancy with the intent of injuring herself as well as destroying the baby.

The Risks of Infection, Hemorrhage and Perforation

I have seen pregnancies terminated by the insertion of a soft catheter into the vagina and up into the uterus. To help the insertion a steel wire has to be put into the catheter. Such a method *does* work, since any foreign object inserted into the uterus may start contractions that will eventually expel the product of a conception. But when the procedure is done by an untrained person who cannot maintain sterile conditions, the dangers of infection are enormous.

The array of objects and substances that have been

inserted into the uterus is almost endless. A generation ago, knitting needles were the standard implements for this form of mutilation. Today's devices, some of which can't possibly ever work, include straightened-out coat hangers, welding cords, Q-tips, and hair pins. You name it and some hapless girl will have already thought of it. If a girl who aborts herself is lucky enough not to become infected, she still runs the risk of starting a flow of blood that she cannot stop. To make matters worse, there is also the danger that the object inserted will perforate the uterus and that the entire peritoneal cavity will become infected.

The Case of Yvonne: An Imported Remedy

Certainly one of the most bizarre cases I have ever witnessed was that of Yvonne, a Frenchwoman in her early thirties. Yvonne, her husband, and their two small girls had recently come to this country, brought here with the help of an aunt, in whose home they lived. One day the aunt, who was a patient of mine, called me in a state of panic. Yvonne was unconscious and bleeding.

I could understand Yvonne's feeling of isolation in a strange land; and since she was surrounded by people whose language she did not speak, it was particularly difficult for her to seek help. But it is significant that even her benefactor aunt had not known that her neice was pregnant.

I soon learned that Yvonne was typical of the withdrawn and potentially suicidal personality; but at the outset of that emergency I had little time to speculate. In Yvonne's bathroom I found a speculum, the instrument a physician uses for a pelvic examination. What was a house-wife doing with a speculum? As I suspected, she had used it to help insert a catheter into her uterus. To compound matters, through that catheter she had forced sweet oil of almond, a time-honored agent in France for self-induced abortion. The oil had entered first the large blood vessels in the wall of the uterus and then the blood stream, and Yvonne had suffered an oil embolism. I rushed her to a hospital, where she remained in a coma for several days. She lost her baby and almost lost her life. The blob of oil circulating through her body reached her brain and eventually her kidneys. She then had a kidney shutdown and we had to rely on a machine to continue that organ's function. It was weeks before I could be sure that Yvonne would survive and months before she recovered.

Another woman was not so lucky: she was already dead when I first saw her. I attended her post mortem at the hospital. She, too, had inserted a catheter into her uterus; then, to help things along, she had hooked a bicycle pump to the catheter and filled her uterus with air. The air had moved up into the large vein that empties blood from the abdominal cavity. There it had been converted into bloody froth, blocking the vessel. The woman had died imme-diately.

There was also a girl who was told by her friends that she could easily clear up her little problem with a perman-ganate douch. Unfortunately, she took their advice, using undissolved tissue-burning permanganate crystals. When I saw her in the hospital emergency room she was almost totally bled out. We transfused her, but no sooner did we get the blood into her veins than it poured out vaginally. She was in such pain that I could not examine her. It was necessary to take her into surgery in order to conduct an examination. I discovered that the crystals had become lodged in the vagina and around the cervix and had burned a hole into a major artery, from which blood was pumping. After the source of the trouble was located, it was relatively simple to tie off the bleeder and save the girl's life. She was, I might add, still pregnant.

Sure-Fire Methods?

Fortunately, many girls who seek to induce their own abortions do not take such great risks. Instead of inserting an object into the uterus, they ingest something that is supposed to cause an immediate miscarriage. To the best of my knowledge, the only ingestible substances—that is, things that you can eat and drink—that do induce an abortion are the heavy metals, such as mercury. They do the job, but they are also lethal.

Almost everything else ingestible is harmless and worthless. Quinine makes the ears ring, but it won't budge the fetus. Castor oil produces a busy time, but it won't affect pregnancy. Pituitary extract, a hormone that induces labor when a woman is close to full term, does little more than produce mild cramps when taken early in pregnancy. Such regional preparations as the turpentine balls taken in the southeastern part of the country are equally ineffective.

Since these approaches to terminating a pregnancy do not work, why are they still used? Why does the myth that they can't fail still persist?

I account for this for two reasons. First, about twelve per cent of all pregnancies, wanted and unwanted, end spontaneously in the first three months. This happens sometimes because the fetus is gravely defective and cannot survive the developmental period, sometimes because of health problems of the mother, and sometimes for reasons we never fully understand. Thus if a woman takes quinine in the hope of ending her pregnancy and a day or so later has a spontaneous abortion—which has nothing to do with the quinine—she will, of course, swear by quinine as a miracle drug for treating unwanted pregnancy.

The second explanation is to be found in the phenomenon of false pregnancy. The quinine or castor oil seems to work and the woman does have a menstrual period, but actually she wasn't pregnant in the first place.

Almost all females feel perfectly competent to diagnose their own pregnancies. In my office a woman will assure me that a baby is on its way because she has never been late before. But few women really have an absolutely regular menstrual cycle. Any number of conditions other than pregnancy can cause a delay in a period or even account for missing several periods. In addition, most of the symptoms of early pregnancy, such as nausea and fatigue, are highly subjective. If a woman *thinks* that she is experiencing them, there is very little that a doctor can do to convince her otherwise. If a doctor tries to explain that a number of emotional factors—remorse, guilt, anxiety and fear—can contribute to a set of vague symptoms that she interprets as pregnancy, the woman simply doesn't hear him. She *knows* that she's pregnant. In fact, false pregnancies, in extreme cases, can persist for a full nine months and can simulate every appearance of a valid pregnancy, but these are not typical.

Still Another Legend

The third method of self-induced abortion, strenuous exertion, also seems to be firmly lodged in our folklore. I have my own theory for this myth. Most doctors are very conscious of the fact that twelve per cent of all pregnant women will lose their babies in their early months of pregnancy, including those eager to carry the babies to full term. To be sure that he will not be blamed if a spontaneous abortion should occur, a doctor will outline for his pregnant patient a careful schedule of what to do and, mostly, what not to do. Many of the restrictions he will place on a patient will have very little scientific basis *unless* a woman is an habitual aborter. Among the restrictions is usually a reasonable limitation of physical exercise.

As a result, this limitation seems irresistible, in reverse logic, to some women seeking self-abortion. If exercise should be avoided to prevent a miscarriage, then the way to bring about a miscarriage is to exercise vigorously. Thus we find women with unwanted pregnancies riding horseback, playing vigorous tennis and taking long mountain hikes. These women may convert themselves into firm-muscled athletes, but they will not dislodge their fetuses simply because of the exercise.

One "let's-get-rid-of-it" technique combines ingestion and exertion. Known popularly as the "gin method," it is scheduled for the time a woman would normally have her menstrual period. She drinks huge amounts of gin, takes a hot bath and then has vigorous sexual intercourse. There is even a specified position for this method: the man enters the woman's vagina from the rear, on the assumption that the angle at which his penis penetrates will facilitate nudging the reluctant fetus to emerge. If this process doesn't work the first time, it is repeated in its entirety: hot bath, gin and sex. This is probably healthy emotional therapy: it doesn't affect the pregnancy, but it makes the participants so euphoric that they stop brooding about it.

Long-Term Damage

In summary, let me restate that self-induced abortion is *the most dangerous way to try to terminate a pregnancy.* It is a very serious risk to life and offers possible permanent impairment. The various short-term threats to health have already been pointed out: hemorrhage, infection and perforation. If any of these occurs and is neglected, complications develop and, ultimately, the patient, if she does not die, becomes a pelvic cripple. The infection may spread to her Fallopian tubes and leave her permanently sterile. She may find herself with painful and widespread damage. She may not be able to have a bowel movement or to urinate without great discomfort and, more often than not, she will find it painful to have intercourse. In most cases, a hysterectomy will eventually have to be performed.

Often, also, psychic damage accompanies the physical damage. The turbulent period of deciding what to do about the unborn child, the stealthy planning to get rid of it, the attempt itself, and the realization that she probably has damaged her health are all likely to contribute toward casting a cold shadow on a woman's sexual responses for the rest of her life.

The Case of Judy: Almost a Pro

No patient I have ever treated seemed as determined to abort herself as twenty-six-year-old Judy, who was brought into my office weak and wan. "Well, doctor," she said as I began the examination, "I guess I've got to take down my shingle."

She told her story quite willingly. She had aborted herself successfully on four previous occasions. A licensed vocational nurse, she had been able, until this last time, to accomplish this with no apparent damage by inserting a catheter into her uterus. This last time, she admitted, she had "really goofed."

I determined that her temperature was 105 and that she had lost about one-half her total supply of blood. Many pints of transfused blood and countless administrations of antibiotics saved Judy's life. When it became clear that a hysterectomy was indicated, I felt that Judy would be separated from an organ that she had already rejected and that she would not be able to use against herself again in the future. It is a frightening thought that even a woman as knowledgeable as Judy, a nurse, did not realize the hazards involved in attempting an abortion without the benefit of the most sterile conditions and the supervision of a doctor skilled in the operation.

These Women Need Help

Many of the grim consequences of a self-induced abortion could be avoided if a woman would seek prompt medical attention at the first evidence of trouble. This evidence, of course, comprises pain, bleeding and fever. Many a woman neglects these symptoms, since she expects some pain and some bleeding as the fetus is expelled. But it is not neglect alone that keeps a woman from a doctor; it is more often an irrational fear that either the physician will stop the miscarriage and the abortion problem will still be there or he will judge the abortion to be illegal—whether it was or it wasn't—and will advise the police. But law enforcement is *not* the doctor's mission. His task is to care for the patient, not to punish or pass judgment on her.

One thing is true of all the women who try to end their pregnancies themselves: they are *determined* to get rid of their babies. The decision for them is not whether or not to have a baby; it is, instead, what method to use to destroy the fetus. These women are so desperate that they see no choice for themselves but to put their health, their future happiness and even their lives on the line. That's their tragedy.

VIII

The Criminal Abortionist

The criminal abortionist is a disappearing breed, but he is making a slow exit. We are in a wry position in America today because abortion is still a crime only for reasons of geography. As long as there are states that either do not permit legal abortions or allow them only for certain women under certain conditions, the pressing need to solve the problem of unwanted pregnancy will be met by the criminal abortionist.

As long as legal restrictions exist on an issue that ought to be entirely between a woman and her doctor—as long as there is legal intrusion in a situation in which *there ought not be a law*—many pregnant women will become lawbreakers. Earlier in this century we created the lethal subculture of the bootlegger by legislating against drinking. We finally extricated ourselves from that irrational disaster by repealing the Prohibition Amendment. In much the same way we, as a society, have created abortion rings, abortion mills, and hole-in-the-wall solo abortion operations. We cannot eliminate these criminal activities by ignoring the need they meet; we can end them only by changing laws that conflict with the public's welfare.

The Right Thing for the Wrong Reason

Almost, any doctor feels a patient's plea for relief deep within him. Dedication and sympathetic understanding make a doctor, to my mind, a better practitioner. It is a soaring sense of power, however, that sometimes traps a doctor into playing a godlike role, and this behavior is particularly disastrous in an unwanted pregnancy situation, wherein a physician's ego may cause him to say yes to an abortion for the wrong reasons.

I remember one such doctor who practiced in a small town in California before liberalization of the abortion law and flaunted the fact that he was breaking the law. He openly disapproved of the restrictions then imposed on abortions and believed that women in need should be helped. Therefore, he had decided that he, standing alone, as he saw it, would render that help. He performed abortions readily and for a very reasonable fee. My chief complaint about him was not that he was an egomaniac but that he was incompetent. A number of his patients were forced to seek postoperative care, and one of these women became a patient of mine. Her uterus had been ruptured and she was badly infected. It took several days in the intensive care unit and thousands of dollars in hospital and medical expenses to save her life.

On a rare occasion a doctor can become involved in illegal abortions because of his own psychosexual problems. One recent instance, widely reported in the press, concerned a very successful and well-regarded Beverly Hills specialist. He certainly wasn't attracted to performing abortions because of the money; his regular practice yielded him an exceedingly high annual income. Instead, he performed abortions as rewards to patients who performed "unnatural sex acts" with him. These desperate women were so in need of abortions that, in order to obtain them, they submitted to the doctor's personal demands.

Another case that made news was that of a benevolent little old lady—not a doctor—who "helped young girls in trouble." She "practiced" in the Midwest and was named "Mother of the Year" by the veterans' organization in her home town. The following year she was arrested, at the age of sixty-eight, because one of her patients died. As far as was known, that was her first fatality in the thirty years that she had done abortions. While this could be considered an enviable record compared to those of other illegal abortionists—and I include a few doctors as well—I most definitely would not place such an individual on my "recommend" list.

The Right Thing for the Right Reason

There was, however, also a doctor in a small religious community in the East who, in his lifetime, did 30,000 abortions. He did them quite openly, for nominal fees, and was a highly respected member of his community. He performed this service out of a deep conviction that it was a humane and sensible solution to a difficult problem, and patients were referred to him by renowned doctors all over the East. In his entire career this doctor lost only one patient, a young woman whose referring physician had not informed him that the patient had a severe cardiac condition. Considering the era in which this doctor practiced, it would not be amiss to call him a hero.

Knowing Less Than Enough

The ominous criminal abortionists are the nonmedical ones. They are usually persons with some links to the medical profession—nurses, technologists, chiropractors and pharmaceutical salesmen—who have direct access to patients. Abortionists who do not have direct access have other contacts such as cabdrivers, bartenders and bell captains. These nonmedical operators have neither the skill nor the equipment to perform an abortion safely or completely. Many do not even maintain aseptic conditions. None has access to a hospital if complications develop.

In a typical criminal abortion performed by someone who is not a doctor, the abortionist uses techniques not unlike those described in the discussion of self-induced abortions. Usually he introduces a foreign object into a patient's uterus, in order to induce uterine cramps, and then does not allow the abortion to conclude on his premises: instead, once the cramps begin, he sends the patient home, or to a friend's home or a motel, where the actual expulsion of the fetus takes place. The patient is thus, more frequently than not, unattended during the most critical phase of the procedure, when she is vulnerable to the complications of hemorrhage, infection and perforation. Such a patient is often the woman who ends up in the hospital emergency room or the coroner's office.

The Case of Audrey: A Woman's Right Doesn't Make Her Right

When an abortion goes wrong, it is not always the fault of the abortionist. Sometimes a woman makes the wrong decision. Audrey is a good case in point.

Audrey, the daughter of divorced parents, had spent her childhood shuttling back and forth between New England and southern California, between a remarried father whose new wife only reluctantly made room for her and an alcoholic mother with a series of short-term lovers, all of whom the little girl was instructed to call Daddy.

Audrey became pregnant at sixteen as the result of an encounter with an older man who apparently typified to her the father who had abandoned her. She fought fiercely to keep her baby, partly to compensate for rejection by both parents and partly to punish them. First she took her newborn baby to her father's home in a conservative Vermont village, but her stepmother made it very clear that Audrey was a fallen woman. Next she brought the baby to her mother's home in Los Angeles, but that didn't work either. Finally Audrey was on her own, working as a waitress to support her son.

After a while Audrey found herself pregnant again. By then she knew that she could not possibly handle the financial and emotional hardships of raising still another child alone. From a friend she obtained the name of a woman who came to her apartment and performed an abortion for a modest fee. Audrey subsequently used the woman's services a second time, still with no ill effects.

Still later a charming and protective older man came into Audrey's life, and so did another pregnancy. Accustomed to thinking of herself as a loser, Audrey never dreamed that her lover would want either her or their baby as a permanent relationship. Assuming that the man saw her in the same demeaning way she viewed herself, she believed that she had no choice but another abortion. But the woman who had served her so well previously could not be found; and so she went to a man she did not know and was charged three times the amount she had paid, to the woman. Three hours after the abortion Audrey was back home, bleeding profusely and in great pain. She reached into the medicine cabinet for something that would make her feel better and came up with a bottle of Seconal. When I saw her in the hospital emergency room she was on the verge of death, not only from the blood loss, but also from the drug overdose.

In order to save her life, I had to sacrifice her potential for future childbearing, and that was particularly unfortunate because the father of her unborn child, who had not been aware of her pregnancy, was deeply in love with her and wanted to get married. They did marry but now they cannot have a family between them. In addition to Audrey's one child, there could have been the one destroyed in the abortionist's office and others in the future. But Audrey had erred—and had altered her future—by not apprising her lover of her condition.

In my practice I always urge a pregnant female to discuss with her parents (if she's a teen-ager) or the man involved her intention to abort. In numerous instances a man is not told of his partner's predicament and therefore loses the opportunity to make known to her that his love is real and that he wishes to have both a child and a lasting relationship.

An Unwanted Legacy

At this point in time, when there is an enormous amount of information available to the public about abortions, criminal abortionists continue to flourish primarily because of the woman's need for secrecy. This need is her unfortunate legacy from society's long-held puritan attitudes. Many a woman with an unwanted pregnancy seems not to realize that she has as much privacy with a doctor for this problem as she has for any other health problem. Whatever she tells her doctor is privileged communication, not to be shared with anyone without her permission. When she enters a hospital for an abortion the procedure that she undergoes must be of public record, but she may use an assumed name if secrecy is a valid issue. Neither a doctor nor a hospital has private investigators to check on patients.

Too often, when she finds out that she is pregnant, the unmarried woman still suffers through a time-honored *but obsolete* ritual: worry, perhaps a few ineffective home remedies, whispered confidences to close friends, furtive phone calls, the agony of indecision, and then, finally, a visit to a criminal abortionist.

If There's No Other Way

Why risk either a criminal abortion or a self-induced abortion when there is the far better solution of a legal abortion? Even a woman with an unwanted pregnancy who lives where legal abortions are not yet available can today avail herself fairly simply of a proper operation. How can she do this? My advice to her is simple and unequivocal: fly, drive or hitchhike to the nearest state where abortions are legally performed.

IX

The Legal Abortion

It ought to be no more complicated for a woman to get an abortion early in her pregnancy than to get a tooth pulled.

It ought to be possible to have the abortion done in a doctor's office, where a skilled professional staff is in attendance and where the patient can have a few hours for recovery. The procedure should be as simple as that.

We've made a great deal of headway in recent years toward this goal, but we remain a long way from attaining it. At the very least we still need abortion procedures that are uniformly legal in every state in the country.

The Twilight Period

Until uniform regulations are developed we will remain in a twilight period that encompasses legal abortions in some states but not in others and a multitude of varying

111

circumstances that permit abortions in the states in which they are allowed.

Unless a woman can have an abortion *upon request*, whatever the personal reasons that convince her she should have one, she continues to be shackled by the judgmental attitudes of the medical profession. Most doctors still do not make abortions easily available, even in the states where they are legal. If a patient comes into a doctor's office with a broken leg from a skiing accident, the doctor mater-of-factly treats the fracture. He might think the patient foolish for risking disability when he did not know how to handle himself properly on skis, but his first concern is restoring the patient to good health. However, a patient who comes in with the consequences of another kind of accident—similarly careless, no doubt, in many instances and who requests what she feels is the proper treatment—in this case, often gets only a disapproving lecture and a discouraging warning. Too often she is forced to walk away from the doctor she knows and has trusted to seek medical attention from a stranger.

Delaying Tactics

In the state in which I practice, abortion laws have been liberalized, but they still require that abortions be done in a hospital. This is an unnecessary requirement, and it works against a troubled woman seeking proper medical help. Most hospitals, particularly the larger ones, are still so encumbered by a rigid committee system that a doctor seeking to admit a patient for an abortion is made to feel that he is engaging in a dubious treatment. The hospital committee, which must approve the doctor's request to perform an abortion, is usually composed of senior staff men who by age and by background tend to be conservative and traditional and are often not at all receptive to today's changing attitudes toward abortion.

Consciously or otherwise, the committee members resort to delaying tactics. Customarily they require that a patient be examined by a psychiatrist, who must determine that her mental health requires that the abortion be performed. This process takes time: it involves an appointment with a psychiatrist, the deliberations of the committee, and the committee's review of the psychiatrist's recommendations. Generally the abortion finally is approved, but by that time the pregnancy has advanced several weeks: in fact, too often it has advanced from one that could have been terminated easily to one whose termination will have to be a major surgical procedure.

Most cases that are presented to a hospital therapeutic abortion committee are approved on psychiatric grounds. In my experience, however, the involvement of a psychiatrist is more frequently than not sheer hypocrisy. Most women seeking abortions are not psychiatrically disturbed and do not need psychiatric consultations, either before or after their abortions. The medical profession, all too characteristically, is merely going through an unnecessary and complicated ritual that does not serve the patients' best interests.

Untangling the Red Tape

Some of us who practice our specialty under these circumstances and who feel very strongly about the right of every woman to make her own decision concerning motherhood have chosen to work at smaller hospitals, which are more flexible and less self-important. I'm at a larger hospital for my general work, but I find it more convenient and less expensive for abortion patients to use smaller hospitals. The abortion committees of smaller hospitals meet every day and, as a rule, accept obstetricians' recommendations without cumbersome red tape. In my relationships with such hospitals I have performed more than 3,000 legal therapeutic abortions since the California law was liberalized in 1967.

I'm, however, required to hospitalize my patients, sometimes for only a few hours, for what could be, in many cases, an office procedure. As a result, patients who more seriously require hospitalization often have to wait for beds, since space is in woefully short supply in most cities. What's more, hospitalization increases the cost of an abortion to a patient, a factor that denies abortions to many of the women who most need them.

How We Do It

Any surgical procedure, even a minor one, is, from the patient's point of view, usually shrouded in mystery. This is particularly true of the abortion, since it has been illegal for so long and is still beclouded by moral and religious considerations.

How is an abortion performed?

The obstetrician has several choices, depending on how advanced the pregnancy is. The most common method in an early pregnancy is the dilation and curettage, commonly referred to as the "D & C." This procedure is performed under a general anesthetic. The doctor dilates or enlarges the cervix, the opening of the uterus. Through this enlarged opening he introduces a special instrument, which extracts the tiny fetus. Then, to be sure that all the tissue related to the pregnancy is removed, he carefully scrapes the entire uterine cavity with a tool called a curette.

Through a newer technique an abortion can now be accomplished with a suction device. In this process the doctor dilates the cervix and introduces a uterine aspirator. This aspirator is connected to a suction pump and, in a matter of a few minutes, it removes the fetal tissue from the uterus. This procedure is vastly easier on the patient than is any other method of terminating a pregnancy. It takes less time and produces a smaller loss of blood. It cannot be used, however, if the pregnancy has advanced beyond twelve weeks, because the fetus at that stage has become too firm.

If We've Waited Too Long

If a pregnancy has gone beyond the fourteenth week—often, inexcusably, because of delays imposed by a hospital committee—the abortion is a more complicated procedure and calls for a longer stay in the hospital. A recently developed technique for such an abortion involves the injection of either a glucose or a salt solution into the amniotic sac in which the fetus is sheltered during pregnancy. This procedure, which is called amniocentesis, can be performed under a local anesthetic. The doctor uses a long needle to pierce the abdominal wall, the wall of the uterus, and finally the amniotic sac. Through the needle the fluid that normally occupies the sac is withdrawn and then a glucose or saline solution is injected. The presence of the foreign solution in the sac ends the developmental process of the fetus within twenty minutes. Approximately twenty-four hours later the patient goes into labor and expels the fetus.

The most extensive procedure for terminating a pregnancy is the hysterotomy, which is a miniature Caesarean section. As is true with women whose babies have been delivered by Caesareans, once this procedure has been used all future pregnancies also have to be delivered by surgical procedure. The hysterotomy usually costs about twice as much as either the D & C or the suction method, and the patient has to remain in the hospital for from three to six days. I usually reserve this method for patients who have requested that they be sterilized, since both procedures can be done at the same time.

A dilemma is often presented by a woman who is just a little too late for the simpler abortion techniques—that is, past her twelfth week of pregnancy—but who is not far enough advanced for the more complex procedures. The major difficulty in performing a simple abortion beyond the twelfth week is that extensive dilation is required to create an opening large enough for the extraction of the firm, large segments of tissue. To help accomplish such an abortion, I use a substance called *laminoria*, a wood product from South America that has the capacity to absorb an enormous amount of water. I insert a small wedge of this wood painlessly into the patient's cervix and leave it in overnight. In the course of that time, the wood expands considerably in size, as a result of absorbing body moisture, and it consequently, with no discomfort to the patient, dilates the cervix. The next day the abortion is a relatively simple procedure.

The Office Is the Place

My method of choice, provided that my patient and I are able to take prompt action to end the pregnancy, is the suction technique that I described above. Since this is a very brief procedure, it is possible for the anesthesiologist on my surgical team to use a new anesthetic agent called ketamine hydrochloride. This drug does not put the patient to sleep; it merely separates her from sensory input: that is, she can hear, see and feel nothing. But her protective body functions continue to operate: she can swallow, cough, sneeze, breathe and protect herself in case she vomits. The effects of the drug wear off gradually, and there is a short period when the patient is partially disconnected from reality. Some patients have described the "coming-to" phase as somewhat psychedelic but have said that this distorted sensation did not last long.

With this minor surgical procedure, which lasts only a few minutes, and this anesthetic agent, which wears off within half an hour, a patient can arrive at the hospital at seven in the morning and, if there are no complications, leave by noon. That allows ample time for preoperative

117

preparation and two or three hours for recovery under a nurse's monitoring.

I have handled approximately 3,000 cases in this manner, and almost every one of them could have been done as safely in my office, where they would have been easier and less expensive for the patients and less wasteful of hospital facilities. *The direction in which a uniform abortion law must move is toward allowing abortions to be performed by qualified physicians in their offices.*

A New Middleman

Today, how does a woman go about having an abortion performed? In some few instances her gynecologist does it himself. I say few instances because most gynecologists are not experienced in this relatively simple procedure. More gynecologists would, I'm sure, perform abortions if they were skilled in abortion procedures. Certainly, with attitudes and laws changing so swiftly, we are going to need more doctors who can perform legal abortions. In some states medical students, as well as increasing numbers of practicing gynecologists, are now learning abortion procedures.

It is presently difficult for a pregnant woman to determine which doctors are willing and able to do abortions. If a patient needs a medical or surgical service, she can telephone the office of her local medical society for the names of three specifically qualified doctors, among whom she can choose. But most communities will not refer her to a doctor for an abortion.

Thus there flourishes a new middleman, the abortion counselor. This quasi-profession originated in the days when virtually all abortions in the U.S. were criminal acts. The middlemen who operated at that time chartered planes and arranged to fly groups of patients to England or Sweden or Japan, where abortions were performed by qualified physicians. Some of those who offered that service were forward-thinking people genuinely concerned with helping women in an impossible plight, but others were simply procurers for foreign abortionists. The service, of dubious legality, was rarely challenged.

Abortion counseling services today advertise their operations openly in metropolitan newspapers and national magazines. Many of them function under the auspices of groups of clergymen or social workers. These services possess lists of qualified doctors in their communities who perform legal therapeutic abortions and they refer patients to these doctors. Money usually changes hands, often in the guise of a donation.

The medical profession, in the past always highly conservative about what it calls "third-party" intervention, has switched its signals since public thinking has increasingly taken the attitude that having an abortion is not a crime. Today the medical profession not only invites third-party intervention in the form of abortion counselors but thrusts such counselors upon its patients. While innumerable women must be profoundly grateful to abortion counselors, and with good reason, it is really ridiculous that these middlemen are needed at all. Just imagine a situation in which a child needing a tonsillectomy could have that operation only if his mother obtained the name of a doctor from a "tonsillectomy counselor"!

119

The Door Is Not Closed

The abortion counselor who actually meets with a prospective patient and discusses with her the implications of her decision performs a very useful function. No woman should be dissuaded from having an abortion; however, it is very important that she fully understands the drastic step she wishes to take. In making her own personal decision, she should have ample opportunity to explore her feelings before she settles on her course of action. If she wishes to share her decision-making with her lover or her husband, she should be advised to do so. If she is legally a minor, she is, of course, required to have parental consent.

A woman should also have the chance to ventilate her feelings in the presence of a trained and objective person, such as her doctor or someone on his staff. If she can talk more openly with her clergyman or her psychotherapist or a social worker, then that person should be her counselor. What is important is that all doors remain open to a patient applying for an abortion until her final committment. I make it particularly clear in the case of a juvenile patient, whose parents might be pressuring her to get rid of her child, that after an open discussion among the girl and her parents and me it is the girl herself who must tell me her decision. No doctor wants to take the child of a pregnant woman who, in her inner heart, really desires to have it.

Is It Murder?

Despite our changing attitudes toward abortion, a number of deeply rooted resistances still block our complete acceptance of it.

Is abortion an act of murder? In the eyes of some religious groups it is. However, since this country is firmly committed to the separation of church and state, I do not believe that anyone's religious convictions, no matter how devoutly held, should be allowed to establish or influence the law of the land. The law does not consider a fetus a legal entity. No death certificate is required when a fetus is aborted.

In our culture, how do we differentiate between an aggregate of animate tissue and a human being? A human being is identified as a recognizable combination of emotional responses, intellectual capacities, and personality traits. The fetus has none of these attributes, except as potentials. Each sperm cell and each ovum has, in a similar sense, the potential of combining with its opposite and forming a human being, yet we don't cry "murder" when these are discharged and literally go down the drain.

I am not an expert concerning the souls of unborn babies, but I have had considerable experience with the physical and psychological well-being of young mothers. I am less concerned with the hereafter than with the here and now, and I think that it is much less murderous to remove a fetus from a woman's uterus than it is to warp the entire life of a young woman who is not ready for motherhood.

Is It Immoral?

Is an abortion conducive to immorality? We live in an age of great sexual freedom, and I believe that the benefits generated by that freedom far outweigh the risks. But let's not delude ourselves into thinking that the delights of sex

121

have been newly discovered by our generation. Sexual experimentation and sexual variety are as old as recorded time, and the fear of pregnancy has not been a very effective deterrent to men and women doing together whatever they want to do. I do not think that either contraceptives or abortions promote promiscuity. I think that the eternal forces of living and loving and, for that matter, dying continue inexorably, outside the reaches of medicine and law and society. The contributions that medicine has made to today's sexual revolution may somewhat diminish fear and guilt and anxiety, but they have not authorized or facilitated a new era of orgies. Sexual freedom originated before the advent of the study of medicine.

Immorality, as I see it, is not defined by either sexual acts or sexual excesses. I can think of few things more immoral than bringing to full term a baby who is not wanted. To subject a defenseless child to neglect, overt or subtle rejection, and sometimes even vindictive brutality is flagrant immorality.

Is It Damaging?

Finally, does an abortion mark a woman psychologically for the rest of her life?

My experience convinces me that the psychological risk of an abortion is vastly overrated. It is astonishing how matter-of-factly most women absorb the experience once it is removed from the cloak-and-dagger atmosphere. To the average patient, the early months of pregnancy do not constitute a lasting emotional experience. She knows that she is pregnant because a doctor has told her so; she may have some slight physical discomfort to provide subjective support for that diagnosis; but, unless she deeply wants or does *not* want her baby, she experiences little permanent emotional change. She is not yet involved with the fetus and has not felt life. She does not identify the fetus as her future baby. Thus if, in the early months, an abortion can be easily arranged and carried out quickly and simply, and if there are no complications, she recovers without a deep sense of loss. Such an abortion, like the brief pregnancy itself, makes very few demands on her, and her recovery is generally swift.

There are exceptions, of course. For a psychiatrically disturbed woman an unwanted baby can be a great hazard to her mental health. At the same time, every experience can become grist for her self-torturing mill. Having sex is traumatic, but not having it is a rejection; being pregnant is threatening, but having an abortion is guilt-producing. Decisions are very difficult to make in cases of emotional disturbance.

The Case of Cecile: The Terror Is Gone

The woman who can make a healthy adaptation to the vicissitudes of living can almost always weather an abortion. I became convinced of this in my experience with Cecile, who first came to me about five years ago. A successful actress of thirty-two, she was married to a man who was a vocational floater. Cecile was the breadwinner in her household. When she faced an unwanted pregnancy she asked me to help her. She simply could not afford to interrupt her career to have a child and raise it. Since there

123

was no way at that time in which I could legally perform an abortion, I put her in touch with people who referred her to a doctor in Mexico.

Cecile was terrified at the prospect of a criminal abortion. She was theatrical enough by temperament to dramatize every aspect of it. The fact that she had to make her arrangements under a false name and meet her abortionist in a clandestine setting compounded her turbulence. After the abortion she developed a rather minor infection and came to me for treatment. She responded well to treatment, but she was so extravagantly keyed up about the abortion that for many months after the infection had been cleared up, she remained very agitated. She was troubled with doubts. Should she have had the baby? Had she damaged her health? Had she endangered her marriage? She was unresponsive to any rational approach. But eventually her sense of crisis subsided and she resumed her career.

Six months ago Cecile came to me and she was pregnant again. Although I could legally do the procedure myself, I had some second thoughts about another abortion for her. However, she was convinced that she did not want a child, so I scheduled her for a therapeutic abortion. The operation was done openly, at a hospital not far from where she lives, by me as her personal physician. The entire procedure was painless, free of complications, and over in a matter of hours. Nonetheless, I braced myself for an emotional aftermath; but it never came. Freed from unnecessary legal entanglements, Cecile had weathered the experience in a rational, routine manner.

124

X

The Male
Partner

The man involved in an unwed pregnancy is not always the villain. Sometimes he may be the victim.

Despite the fact that my patients all are women, I see more reputed fathers than one might suspect. Sometimes a man doubts a girl's claim that she is pregnant and asks me to examine her to verify it, but more often a man comes to my office with his mate not as her adversary but to give her emotional as well as financial support.

The man who gets an unmarried woman pregnant is not always indifferent to the situation or irresponsible concerning its consequences. I know that a man has a natural impulse to walk away from the problem of an unwanted pregnancy, but I think that most girls, too, would walk away from such a pregnancy if it were biologically possible to do so. With an unexpected pregnancy, if an abortion is easily obtainable, both the man and the woman usually prefer to arrange for one.

The Legal Limbo

The legal rights of the putative father are extremely tenuous. If he marries the child's mother, he assumes the rights and responsibilities of a father, including full financial responsibility for the child. Short of marriage, he is nowhere. He is no part of the decision of whether or not the mother will have the child aborted; nor does he have any say in whether or not she will place the child for adoption. Furthermore, he is often in a potentially hazardous position, subject to criminal action on rape charges or to civil action in a paternity suit. By tradition, society assumes that the male is a defiler of innocence and that the female needs all the protection that the legal system can muster for her.

I have seen many cases in which I thought that this protective attitude was well warranted, but I have also seen instances in which it was misplaced. I have known many a man who did not know about an abortion until after it had taken place and who would have preferred that the child be born. I have also known many a man who went to great trouble and took considerable legal risks to arrange a criminal abortion, drove the mother of his child to Mexico, paid for her abortion, and took care of her while she recovered.

Now that legal abortions are possible in my practice, many putative fathers accompany their mates on the first visit to see me as patients, bring them to the hospital, and support them in every sense of the word. Many out-of-state women also arrive at my office for help, and they, too, are rarely alone. In fact, I can safely say that I see more men in my office who are concerned and responsible participants in an illegitimate pregnancy than I do husbands of women to whom I am giving routine prenatal care.

While a man may sometimes be the victim of an illegitimate pregnancy that has been engineered in order to trap him into marriage, the reverse is also true: sometimes a man maneuvers a woman into marriage. In either case, pregnancy is a bad ploy. Marriage is a rough enough course without the handicap of an unwanted child.

The Case of Jerry: A Warped Future

Rough as is the marriage course, I frequently discover a stubborn responsibility toward it in youngsters who are very much a part of today's world. Jerry is the son of a friend of mine, an upper-middle-class suburban lawyer. Jerry suffers from the complete syndrome of alienation: he is distressed about the world in which he lives, contemptuous of the establishment, uncomfortable about himself, and seeking self-identification in varied ways. He dropped out of college and left home at nineteen, found solace of sorts in drugs, and joined a large, communelike household with a group of like-minded youngsters, including a beautiful girl from India.

When Jerry's girl became pregnant he married her, and I delivered their baby boy. The advent of his son was a turning point in Jerry's life. He took stock of himself and

127

decided that the world he wanted for his son did not include stoned parents. His first step at self-reclamation was to get off drugs. His father was tremendously supportive and, with the aid of some psychotherapy, Jerry became unaddicted. His wife, however, was not so lucky.

Jerry was profoundly torn. He loved his wife and son, but he was afraid that if he stayed with them he would slip back into drug use. If he left them, there was a reasonable chance for his return to college and his ultimately becoming a better-equipped breadwinner and father. Reluctantly he moved out, leaving his son behind. He is now living with his parents and going to school part time. What he earns at a part-time job he sends to his wife for the baby. But he remains tormented. Although he is clearly on his way up once again, he feels that he has made the wrong decision in terms of his child. He feels sure that the money he sends to his wife is often spent on drugs instead of food. He knows that his wife is less and less attentive to the needs of their child. Jerry is alternately angry, resentful and remorseful. His parents will probably rescue their grandson soon and bring him to their home for rearing. In this case, it is the father, not the mother, whose future life is being warped by an illegitimate pregnancy.

Whose Responsibility?

I do not mean to present the man in an illegitimate pregnancy invariably as a hero nor do I present him as a martyr. It is just that I know that more men behave responsibly than is commonly believed and I bear in mind the fact that the responsibility for avoiding pregnancy has largely shifted from the male to the female.

Once the primary contraceptive was the condom. Today it's the pill. *She* takes the pill: *she* makes the decision of whether or not to risk pregnancy. Often, in fact, a woman is reluctant to let her mate know that she is pregnant. I have had many a young patient who stubbornly refused to tell either me or her parents the identity of the man responsible for her pregnancy because she felt that the pregnancy was her fault and therefore did not want the man burdened with the situation.

There is no way to predict how either partner will react to or get through the problem of unplanned parenthood. I have seen both partners suffer, often disproportionately. I have seen both behave with indifference, resentment, duplicity and cruelty. And, on many rewarding occasions, I have seen both conduct themselves with courage, grace and tenderness.

XI

Liberating
the Married Woman

The plight of the pregnant unmarried woman is poignant and usually dramatic and often calls for a tortured decision. But the truth is that more abortions are performed on married women than on single women. In fact, even greater numbers of married women will undoubtedly choose to have abortions in the future.

Most married women decide not to have children in consultation with their husbands, and their reasons are usually entirely practical and rational. Thus for them the procedure of abortion is infinitely less conspiratorial and shame-ridden than it is for single girls. Among the most compelling reasons for not having a child is the feeling that the family is complete with its present number of children. What the father and mother can afford becomes a consideration with those who wish to provide a decent standard of living and who realize that a comfortable home and proper nutrition, medical care and educational opportunities cannot realistically be distributed among more and more children without decreasing the advantages to each child. I personally do not believe that sacrifices should be imposed on some children for the sake of others. Children, after all, have no choice about whether or not their family continues growing.

Parents also sometimes decide not to bring to full term a life they have inadvertently started because of emotional economy. Meeting the emotional needs of sons and daughters becomes increasingly taxing as children respond demandingly, and often chaotically, to today's stressful environment. Devoted and responsible parents strive to be always available to their children, alert to their incipient problems, and able to give them sensitive support and guidance. Few parents have an unlimited emotional reservoir from which to draw, and if they spread themselves too thin, someone is inevitably deprived.

The Case of Maggie: Not Enough to Go Around

Maggie thinks of herself as the ideal mother, and she has twelve children to prove it. An only child, Maggie was always aware of her mother's sense of inadequacy at not surrounding Maggie with brothers and sisters. Maggie was determined that her family life would be different, and she and her husband, both Catholic, decided to have a large family.

Maggie has been my patient for years, and some of her

131

older children are now my patients too. Money is not a problem, because Maggie's husband is adequately successful, and Maggie denies her youngsters nothing. Even so, there is not a happy child in the family. Maggie tries to divert the children with food, so most of them are gravely obese. Among the older ones, those who are not on diet pills are experimenting with mind-bending drugs. There is enough of everything in that home *except perceptive attention to the individual needs of each child*. Maggie has overextended herself in terms of her emotional resources. As a result, her children, though indulged in some ways, are deprived in others.

The American woman today is far more realistic than she was years ago about her life after her children are grown. A generation or two ago, some mothers whose children no longer needed their incessant attention often were overwhelmed with a sense of uselessness. Such women sometimes sought refuge in menopausal doldrums, alcoholism, or nervous breakdowns. Today, most women anticipate their children's independence and prepare for it. Some of my patients have returned to college or have taken vocational training for a new career or have joined their husbands in business ventures. Some of these women have had very little previous work experience and have enjoyed the challenge of testing themselves in new settings. Others, who have interrupted stimulating careers in order to raise families, have wanted to contribute to society by returning to teaching or nursing or social work.

For a woman who has already raised a family and is seeking new goals, an unplanned pregnancy can be a particularly damaging psychological blow. It is also often ill-advised medically for an older woman to become pregnant, since children born of mothers over forty run a higher risk of being congenitally damaged. In almost all instances of pregnancy in an older woman, the best course to follow is abortion.

The Case of Arlene: A Second Blooming

Abortion is the choice that I was able to offer to Arlene. At forty-seven she and her husband had two children, who were both grown, married, and on their own. When she had finished college as a young adult, Arlene had worked as an apprentice dress designer and had shown a very promising talent. Five years ago she opened a small business in order to design and manufacture women's fashions. The firm flourished from the start, but it required constant attention. Arlene was totally absorbed in her work, and both she and her husband were elated at her enjoyment of this second blooming. She was lively, involved, and receiving enormous satisfaction from her sense of achievement.

Then she became pregnant. She had mistakenly assumed that she was in her menopause and had felt no further need for contraceptives. Her whole exciting new world seemed about to topple, and the burdens of taking care of a newborn, at her age, appeared overwhelming. All too well she could remember the night feedings, the incessant changings and bathings and burpings, and the sense of being housebound. All these things had been a joy when she was younger, and she had done them willingly and

133

lovingly. But she didn't want to do them again. For both Arlene and her husband, an abortion was the civilized and humane solution.

The Case of Beth and Allen: No More Blighted Babies

For some couples I have absolutely no doubts: nothing but an abortion will do. The woes that had descended upon Beth and Allen led me readily to that conclusion. These two people, both twenty-three, seemed to be born losers. Although they were so young, when I first met them Beth had already given birth to five children. First she had had twins: one had died and the other was mentally retarded. Then, heartbreakingly, a son had been born blind. By that time, Beth and Allen should have been amply warned that either one or both of them was blighted by a grave genetic defect. But not a soul apparently had given them the candid counseling that they had needed as they floated along in the happy dream of having a large family. As a result another pregnancy produced another set of twins, both of whom were mentally retarded.

It was during her next pregnancy that Beth became my patient. She and Allen had at last come to the realization that she could not possibly cope with another baby, considering the needs of the present houseful of handicapped children. They also couldn't face the prospect of Beth's being delivered of another abnormal infant. At the request of both parents I performed an abortion and, in addition, sterilized Beth. I cannot contend that I have solved this couple's overwhelming problems, but I have certainly prevented further problems from developing.

The Case of Laura: Not a Home-Wrecker

A mature woman who has been engaged in extramarital sex will usually seek an abortion to protect her own marriage, but Laura, a forty-two-year-old childless widow, wanted to protect the marriage of the man with whom she was involved.

Laura was the secretary to the administrator of a large metropolitan hospital, where she met Les, a black physician on the hospital staff. She had been a virgin at marriage and had had no sexual activity during her twelve years of widowhood. But with Les, Laura was deeply moved sexually. Les was also sexually aroused by Laura, despite the fact that he was married and had five children.

One night the inevitable happened and, like many women who have never been pregnant, Laura gave little thought to preventing conception.

Part of Laura must have wanted very much to have Les' child, but that was out of the question. If she gave birth to a child of mixed racial heritage, rearing it herself would confront her with more problems than she felt she could manage. Furthermore, since almost the entire hospital staff knew that Laura and Les had a close and warm friendship, the appearance of a black baby at the conclusion of Laura's pregnancy would almost certainly destroy Les' marriage. To prevent these problems, the obvious answer was an abortion.

The Case of Edna and Gene: Scrap the Marriage or Save It?

Edna, on the other hand, salvaged her own marriage by an abortion. Edna and Gene were the very embodiment of all the myths about a romantic love. Childhood sweethearts, "steady" dates by the time they were in their mid-teens, and deeply in love, they were married as soon as they finished high school. At that time both were virgins. Through the years they had a full and rewarding marriage, and their three children, now in their teens, are delightful youngsters who are full of promise and are well prepared by their parents for the independence they will soon embark upon.

Three years ago Edna and Gene decided, after a great deal of soul-searching discussion, that they were sure that they had as large a family as they wanted. To make certain that they would have no additional children, Gene had a vasectomy.

A year ago, Edna, restless because the children needed little mothering, got a part-time job as a checker in a supermarket. Paul, the store's assistant manager, was attracted to Edna, but she dismissed his attentions lightly: she had heard that women who work *expect* their bosses to make at least verbal passes at them.

However, what Edna could not dismiss was her long-suppressed curiosity about what it would *really* be like to go to bed with someone other than her husband. Edna found that she was daydreaming about it, that her sleep was haunted by it, and that her relationship with her husband was tainted by it. She finally decided to find out, and before long, scarcely accustomed to the role of unfaithful wife, she realized that she was pregnant.

One thing was abundantly clear: there wasn't a chance in the world of convincing Gene that the child was his. The more she thought about her predicament, the firmer became her decision that she didn't want to deceive Gene further. She quit her job without telling Paul that she was pregnant and that evening confessed the entire episode, pregnancy and all, to Gene. Together they reviewed their life and discussed the life that lay ahead for them. To Gene there was no doubt that what they had was far too valuable to be scrapped because of one mistake. He was, it seemed to Edna, almost saintly in forgiving her. But he was not so saintly as to want to raise another man's child, and they agreed that Edna should not have the baby.

Edna and Gene were fortunate: when their love was tested, it turned out to be stronger than either of them thought.

The New Face of Freedom

Freedom for today's married woman extends beyond her new capacity to decide whether or not to have an unwanted child. She is free, too, to seek variety in her sexual experiences without abandoning her marriage and, often, without jeopardizing it. I don't know whether more married women are having extramarital affairs now than twenty years ago, but I do know that more of them are talking openly about their activities to their friends, their doctors and sometimes—if it suits their purposes—even to their husbands.

Sexual adventuring is done sometimes out of curiosity, sometimes in retaliation, sometimes because it is "the thing to do," and sometimes because a husband encourages his wife to experiment with other men. An affair develops sometimes from overwhelming sexual attraction. One relationship may start as love and another may end as love. Such an interlude for a wife need not threaten a marriage any more than the occasional dalliance of a husband inevitably threatens it. In fact, if a woman is adroit, discreet, and not tormented by guilt, an affair may even save her marriage.

The Case of Carol: Sex as a Lifesaver

In the case of Carol an affair literally saved a life. Carol's husband, Archie, is a very successful writer. Seven years ago, when he was forty-nine, he had a massive heart attack and just barely recovered. He became a cardiac cripple and was warned that any physical exertion would endanger his life.

Sexually speaking, Carol and Archie were finished. During the first few months of Archie's convalescence, Carol was so grateful to have Archie alive that she assured herself, and him, that sex was immaterial. Carol then was thirty-eight, very lovely and very active, and she misjudged her own sex drive. Archie, however, was wise enough to perceive it, and they had what must have been an extraordinarily frank discussion, laden with devotion. Archie insisted that Carol's sexual needs to fulfilled.

Although they had no children, they were realistic enough to admit that pregnancy might be a consequence of Carol's adventuring; but that was a consequence that neither of them would welcome. They came to see me together and told me of their dilemma and how they wanted to resolve it. I put Carol on the pill.

Since that time, Carol has had a sex life that she has

managed with the utmost discretion and in privacy. Archie never knows what Carol is doing; nor does he press her to tell him who she sees. Carol seems happy, and Archie is happier than he would be if he were holding his wife a prisoner of his illness. This arrangement has continued for seven years. It is a civilized solution for a desperate problem.

The Case of Helen: New Route to Motherhood

We tend to think of sexual freedom in terms of escape: having sex without getting pregnant or getting pregnant but not have a baby. To Helen, sexual freedom meant, instead, the ability to make sure of becoming pregnant and having a baby.

Helen and Dave are friends as well as patients of mine. Dave is quite an authoritative man, a bank manager, successful and accustomed to having his way. Helen and Dave had a happy marriage, but after eight years they were still childless. I think that this situation was particularly bitter for Dave since he felt responsible after he learned from a urologist that his sperm count was low.

Helen, too, was unhappy about their inability to have children. She believed that it threatened their marriage. She also felt called upon constantly to reassure Dave about his masculinity. One day she came to talk with me about the possibility of pregnancy through artificial insemination. I explained the process involved in getting viable sperm from a donor. She listened carefully, musingly, and said that she would think about what I had told her. She also said that she had not yet discussed artificial insemi-

139

nation with her husband. My own unspoken feeling was that Dave would never consent.

About six months later, Helen came to see me again; this time she was triumphantly pregnant. She had convinced herself that if she was going to have a baby with another man's sperm, she might as well do it naturally rather than artificially. She had carefully considered who might be the best prospect and had finally settled for a man in her neighborhood who had three beautiful children. Their deal had been this: as much sex as they wanted and needed until she got pregnant, at which time they would be through with each other.

Dave has never doubted that the child is his. He believes that his doctor made a mistake: that's what he thought all along, and now his feeling has been confirmed. Helen went through the entire experience with magnificent tranquility. She has her little boy, she has a happy husband, and she has preserved a good marriage. And both Helen and Dave smile appreciatively when their friends tell them, as good friends invariably do, that little Davie looks exactly like his daddy.

In today's vocabulary, Arlene, Beth, Carol and Helen all chose their own forms of liberation. New medical advances may have played a role in their choices, but that role was minor. The moving force in each choice was the personal courage of the individual woman. A social climate that encourages such open self-honesty is, in my opinion, the major contribution of the sexual revolution.

XII

The Right Way
to Have a Baby

If a woman decides to have a baby, that baby will be born into a world that is rough and tough. That world will make exacting demands on the mind and body of the new person she has formed, so the least she can do is give it a good start.

It is not difficult to give an unborn child a safe and nourishing environment, and most women competently do so. Widespread health information is available in the schools, in magazines and books, and on television. Medical science's numerous dramatic advances have reduced some of the more somber risks that once accompanied pregnancy. In addition, the thinking of many doctors has changed considerably: we no longer view pregnancy as a span of time dominated by a series of "don'ts." Instead, we urge a healthy young woman, unless she has obvious complications, to go through her pregnancy casually and to live in her usual style.

What I state in this chapter about having a healthy baby is not intended to serve as a manual for prenatal care. A pregnant woman will receive detailed instructions from her doctor and should follow them. If she has pre-existing health problems or her condition suggests the possibility of complications, her doctor may stress elements of care quite different from those I am about to set forth. A woman should listen to her own doctor, not to me.

Just as I believe that *not* having an unwanted baby is part of a woman's rightful choice today, so do I believe that *having* a baby means that a woman will be responsible for favoring it with all possible initial opportunities.

Changing Eating Habits

The one element that I usually change in a patient's normal routine is her diet. This is particularly true if she's still in her teens and is ingesting too many carbonated drinks and starchy snacks and too much candy. A pregnant woman must have a diet high in protein, and two-thirds of her protein requirement should be supplied by such animal-protein foods as meat, eggs, cheese, poultry and fish, since these are the foods that supply the essential amino acids. The remaining protein requirement of a pregnant woman can be supplied from such vegetable-protein foods as beans, peas, and cereals of whole grains, especially wheat.

A sound diet at any period of life should include protein, and during pregnancy the intake of protein foods should be increased by *at least fifty per cent*. Ordinarily a full-grown woman needs very little in the way of building material, except to repair damaged tissue; but during pregnancy she engages in a tremendous building task, in order to have a bigger uterus, bigger breasts, more blood, and a placenta for nourishing the fetus. All of this expansion requires protein, the substance that is essential to the adequate physical development of the baby. In recent years we have determined that the child who is undernourished during his prenatal months is likely to be stunted mentally as well: his brain may not develop adequately, his learning ability may be impaired, and his capacity to adapt to life may be reduced.

Who runs the greatest risk of producing a protein-deprived baby? One person is an impoverished mother who cannot afford the food she needs and thus forces her baby to start life badly equipped to cope with the disadvantaged environment into which he is born. Another person is a young woman from the "hippie" world who may be a food faddist and may shun most of the protein-rich foods. Even though nuts and other meat substitutes provide some protein, they do not supply anywhere near enough. Finally, there is, in some circles, an abnormal value placed on being thin. Generally speaking, I consider a lean patient a better health risk than an obese one, but not if it means starving an unborn baby.

The Case of Roberta: She Starved Her Baby

Self-starvation and consequent fetal starvation are not limited to cultists, but I did not expect to find those conditions in Roberta, a physiotherapist.

143

At age thirty-two Roberta was tough, wiry, not the most seductive of women, and one who had very little sexual experience. She was gifted with patients, quite scholarly in her approach to her profession, and as interested in research as in clinical experience. Her predominant drive was to get ahead in her career. When the subject of sex was mentioned in her conversations with co-workers, she dismissed it rather abruptly; sex, she was convinced, could wait until she was married.

However, a new orthopedic surgeon at the hospital completely changed her attitude. He was married but in the process of getting a divorce. He and Roberta shared a dedication to their work. Together they made a very resourceful pair of healers. Their mutual admiration for each other was apparent to all. The attraction soon deepened into love, and Roberta, the perennial scoffer at sentimental attachments, happily embarked on an affair.

When she told her lover that she was pregnant he replied in no uncertain terms that he had no intention of ever marrying again. I was dismayed at the deep depression that engulfed Roberta. Just as she had blossomed into radiance with the advent of love, she seemed to wither under the impact of disappointment and rejection. She became perilously withdrawn and, despite all my attempts to persuade her to safeguard her health, she refused to eat. A thin woman normally, she lost six pounds during her pregnancy.

Roberta carried her baby to full term and was delivered uneventfully of a five-and-one-half-pound son who seemed to be normal. She placed him for adoption.

Now once again totally immersed in her career, Roberta insists that she is through with men forever and, to all appearances, seems happily adjusted. Her son, however, has not fared as well. The family who adopted him assumed that he was normal, but gradually, over the past five years, this family has had to accept the fact that the boy is developing slowly, a persistently below-average child. There is no way that I can prove that Roberta's self-starvation was the cause of her baby's slow rate of development, but my experience with this particular patient—as well as with others who refuse or neglect to eat proper foods—has reinforced my conviction that good nutrition is crucial to a healthy pregnancy.

Vitamins? No Big Deal

Can pregnant women make up for dietary neglect with vitamins? I'm afraid that I must puncture this misconception that, I'm sorry to say, has been perpetrated by many doctors as well as by vendors of vitamins. Most women, pregnant or otherwise, do not need vitamins. During pregnancy, they usually need supplementary iron and calcium. All of them, however, seem to feel neglected if they are not instructed to take vitamins. Vitamins mistakenly—and unfortunately—give patients the assuring feeling that they are taking good care of themselves. Therefore, most doctors, myself included, satisfy their expectations by reciting the usual instructions about consuming those supplementary pellets. Vitamins do women no harm unless they mislead themselves into thinking that they can bypass the natural protein they need.

145

Let's Not Go Overboard

The effect of drugs on fetal development is still, for the most part, a great unknown, and doctors today tend to be cautious in prescribing medication for pregnant patients. There is, for example, evidence that the use of tranquilizers and antidepressants during pregnancy *may* sometimes arrest the development of a child, making him a slow learner. All doctors know that almost any medication powerful enough to help a patient is also powerful enough to have the potential for damaging her as well. We must therefore, for each patient, weigh the benefits against the hazards. For a woman to be told to renounce all medication, even aspirin, during pregnancy is preposterous. I'm confident that I serve both the mother and the fetus best by putting an agitated mother on tranquilizers, when necessary, so that she will remain calm enough to carry her baby to full term. Further, if I recognize a patient as being probably suicidal, I would rather take the calculated risk involved in prescribing antidepressants than the much greater risk of her possibly satisfying her self-destructive drive and ending not only her life but also her baby's.

How Drugs Damage Babies

Drugs that are medically indicated should be judged quite differently from drugs taken purely for kicks. While not all mind-expanding drugs have been demonstrated to be harmful, not one of them helps the pregnant woman in the least and many of them do predictable damage.

Let's consider the least harmful substances first. Neither marijuana nor alcohol seems to affect fetal development, but extreme users of either are usually indifferent to good eating habits and are often prone to accidents and injuries. Therefore, in the long run, marijuana and alcohol are likely to inflict indirect damage on babies.

Now let's discuss the harder drugs. There is already firm evidence of damage from some of them, and the suspicion is growing that they may do even greater harm than we have as yet been able to prove. Heroin is unquestionably damaging during pregnancy: users have a high rate of prematurity and their babies have lower birth weights and reduced chances for survival. If a mother withdraws from heroin prior to delivery, the fetus will not be addicted at the time of birth; but if she is on heroin at the time of delivery—information she rarely shares with her obstetrician—the baby will be born addicted.

If you have never watched a newborn go through withdrawal symptoms, you are fortunate. It's a shocking, dismaying and heart-rending sight. The puny, pasty-looking infant may have convulsions; it is weak and jittery; and there is recent experimental evidence that it experiences severe pain during withdrawal.

Though the acute phase of this disorder may last only a few days, the baby who is an addict at birth will not eat properly, further damaging his chances for survival. In fact, this feeding problem may persist for a month or so. Usually born prematurely, such an infant has forced upon it burdens that are almost too staggering for him to cope with.

There also seems to be a strong indication that the use of LSD causes chromosomal damage. We are not yet in a position to say positively that LSD directly causes fetal abnormality, but there is already enough of a basis for the suspicion that this conclusion will be correct. If our medical suspicions are well founded, a young woman on LSD—or any other drug, for that matter—must do her utmost, with her doctor's help, not to indulge her habit once she finds out that she is pregnant.

The most profound damage done to a fetus, either from drugs or from infection, occurs during the first three months of its development, when all of its vital structures are in the process of formation. Often a woman does not even realize that she is pregnant until she is almost through that crucial period in her pregnancy. When that happens to a drug user, the discovery comes too late to spare the fetus from possible damage.

Panic Doesn't Help

I have had young patients tell me defiantly that there is little purpose in safeguarding their internal health when they are forced to live in an external environment whose air, water, and food are contaminated. I concede that pollution is a grave problem and that it may well be determined that some of the contaminants actually inflict fetal damage. But that possibility, over which the individual pregnant woman has little control, fails to jusitfy the neglect of her own personal health, over which she has considerable control.

Pollution, it is agreed, is a threat that we must not ignore. As a nation we *are* taking countermeasures. But no purpose is served by exaggeration or by panicking the populace. The supersalesmanship that characterizes so much of American life—for good as well as bad—is driving full force to alert people to the dangers of contamination. But announcing, for example, that mother's milk is so laden with DDT that if it were a commercial product it would never pass government inspection is only making a gross overstatement that serves no useful purpose. Millions of babies are fed their mothers' milk and thrive on it. Undoubtedly a mother and baby in a heavily polluted area would fare better in a brighter, cleaner environment, but their prospects are not improved by the mere telling of horror stories.

Will a Baby Be Defective?

For many a woman, pregnancy is haunted by the possibility that she will give birth to a malformed baby or one who will be blighted by a lifelong illness. Such babies are born each day, and we can't always explain what went wrong. But in many cases we do understand the causes of congenital defects. Fortunately, we are able to do more today to stave off these catastrophes than we were even as recently as ten years ago. Some defects we can now prevent. Others we can detect early enough in fetal life to abort a hopelessly defective baby.

We now have methods available that can almost eliminate the disaster of the Rh baby, the one whose blood type is incompatible with his mother's. This antagonism between the two blood types rarely affects the woman's first child but often threatens future children. The disorder may result in a stillborn baby, a mentally retarded child, or

149

an infant so anemic that only a complete exchange trans-
fusion will save its fragile life. These days a serum can be
given to the mother within seventy-two hours after the
birth of the first baby—and of each subsequent baby—that
will protect a succeeding infant from the risks of the Rh
factor.

Goodbye to German Measles

On another front of medical science we seem to be on
the threshold of wiping out German measles, or rubella. As
a disease of childhood, German measles is mild and harmless. As a disease of a woman in her early months of pregnancy, it produces a high risk that a seriously damaged
baby will result. The pregnant woman who develops German measles almost always catches it from one of her own
children or a child in the neighborhood. Today a new vaccine is being given to children so that they will no longer
primarily endanger pregnant women.

It might be logical to ask why we do not vaccinate
pregnant women. The reason we do not is not so simple.
Most women have had German measles as children, and
they are safe from a second affliction. But the ones who
have never been afflicted can be infected by the vaccine—
as can their fetuses—whether they are vaccinated during
pregnancy or during the few months preceding pregnancy.

It is now possible to tell by blood tests, however,
whether or not a woman has ever had German measles.
Those who test negative must, of course, be watched carefully. Though a patient may test negative at the start of
her pregnancy, a few weeks later she may develop symp-

toms that might or might not mean an infection of German measles. In that case, I test her blood again, and if her test changes to positive I have to tell her that she faces a very real risk of producing a defective baby. At that point she may choose to bypass the risk by having an abortion.

Life-or-Death Decisions

Perhaps the most dramatic break-through in my specialty in recent years has been the development of a process called amniocentesis, by which we are able to tell a number of things about a baby long before its birth. This process, which can be carried out as early as the fourteenth or fifteenth week of pregnancy, involves inserting a needle through a woman's abdominal wall and into the amniotic sac in order to draw out a portion of the amniotic fluid. The withdrawn fluid is then subjected to a chromosomal analysis, which reveals, among other things, the sex of the unborn infant and the presence or absence of certain diseases. Such information often serves as the basis for life-or-death decisions.

The Case of Butch and Lynn:
The Odds Were Not in Their Favor

I used this dramatic means of diagnosis to help Butch and Lynn reach a crucial decision. Before Lynn became my patient they had had one baby, a tragically afflicted child who had died shortly after birth as the result of what is known medically as Down's syndrome and more commonly as Mongolism. The disease is a grim experience for parents, but it does not usually occur twice in the same

151

family. Statistically, it occurs in one of every 2,000 births but rarely happens more than once to the same mother and father. There are, however, many forms of Down's syndrome and one rare type is very much more threatening. This medical rarity, called DG translocation, works as follows: if three babies are born into a family afflicted with the disease, one baby will be normal, one will be normal but a carrier—that is, he will transmit the defect to the next generation—and one will be afflicted. If but one child is born to parents with the disease, it can turn out to be any of the three types: normal, a carrier, or abnormal.

Before Lynn's baby had died, a chromosomal analysis of its blood had revealed that the disorder carried in the parents' genetic endowment was DG translocation. But since Butch and Lynn wanted desperately to have a family, they decided to take a chance on another pregnancy. It was early in this pregnancy that Lynn became my patient. Understandably, she was having second thoughts, very worried and disturbed thoughts, about having her child. I immediately did an amniocentesis and discovered that the fetus was indeed afflicted with the disorder. As a result, Lynn, her husband and I promptly decided upon a therapeutic abortion.

But now that Lynn was aware she could know in advance if she was going to have an abnormal baby and could take corrective measures, she decided to become pregnant again. Once more I checked the fetal cells early in the pregnancy, and this time the cells tested normal; the fetus was neither afflicted nor a carrier. The little boy is the only baby they'll ever have, but they are thankful. The odds were not in their favor, but medical advances and liberalized legal procedures helped them to produce what they wanted: a normal child of their own.

The Case of Rachel: Escape from Doom

Rachel had her first child early in her marriage. When she became my patient, that son, Jimmy, was fifteen. He had hemophilia, a hereditary disease in which it is virtually impossible to control bleeding. During his young life, Jimmy had spent about two months out of every year in the hospital. His mother, who loved him dearly, had died a thousand deaths with each of his bleeding episodes.

When Rachel came to see me, she was in the third month of a new pregnancy. She stated that she couldn't attempt raising another child with problems as devastating as Jimmy's. She had decided upon an abortion. As I talked with her I realized that she really wanted the baby she was carrying. I also realized that she was unaware that hemophilia, though a hereditary disease, does not inevitably reoccur. It is sex-linked and is characteristically passed on from a mother to half of her sons; it is very rare for a baby girl to be afflicted. When I explained this to her she eagerly consented to amniocentesis. Happily, we learned that she was carrying a little girl.

When Rachel had her baby not only her outlook on life but also Jimmy's changed: the family no longer thinks of itself as doomed.

The Permissive Pregnancy

Most pregnancies, of course, are not as dramatic as the cases I have discussed. Most are relatively simple matters of day-to-day living, of growing and hoping and planning.

There are very few prohibitions that I issue flatly to my pregnant patients. Most women can live reasonably active lives. I encourage those who are working to hold their jobs for as long as they comfortably can. The days when pregnancy was a period of enforced invalidism are gone, except for special cases. The woman who habitually aborts, for instance, may need to spend her entire pregnancy at bed rest, and the same may be true for the woman who is carrying twins; but most women should be encouraged to enjoy their pregnancies by doing what comes naturally.

It is not necessary to cancel travel plans. Most travel today is done by plane, and nothing about the average flight threatens a pregnancy. At one time we were reluctant to have our patients travel because we feared that they might develop unanticipated complications in remote areas where good medical attention was unavailable. But today almost every major city in the world has well-trained obstetricians to whom a patient in distress can be directed.

The edict against bathing and douching during pregnancy is outmoded, too. The only hazard connected with bathing arises in the later months, when the woman tends to be somewhat clumsy and hence is more likely to slip and fall. Douching is often particularly helpful when a woman is pregnant. Since she commonly develops vaginal discharges, douching will contribute to her comfort. My only warning about this cleansing process is to avoid running water into the vagina with excessive force.

Can a woman have sexual intercourse during pregnancy? Why not? For one thing, pregnancy should not be a period of deprivation. For another, many couples experience extraordinary feelings of tenderness toward each other at this time that they wish to and should express sexually. Many a man derives specific erotic stimulation from the sight of his full-breasted pregnant wife and is at his best sexually during her pregnancy. My instructions to my patients are simple: as long as both the husband and the wife are comfortable, *physically and psychologically*, they can safely continue sexual intercourse. Only if the act becomes a problem to *either of them* should it be discontinued.

There is one point at which my customary permissiveness stops, however. I do not want my patients to smoke. That's right. I don't want them to smoke. I know, however, that many smokers won't quit; but I do insist that they reduce their habit during pregnancy. There is a good reason for this insistence: a pregnant woman who smokes heavily increases her chances significantly of having a spontaneous abortion early in pregnancy. In addition, a smoker tends to have respiratory problems that may complicate her pregnancy. Additionally, statistically babies born to heavy smokers tend to be underweight at birth.

Natural Childbirth: Pro and Con

The exciting and dramatic culmination of pregnancy is the delivery of the child. Despite the hundreds of times I have taken part in childbirth, the process never ceases to amaze and thrill me.

Many of my patients today are choosing to deliver through natural childbirth—that is, without the aid of anesthesia or any pain-relieving medication. If a woman feels that she can manage it and if her motivations are honest, I think that natural childbirth is all to the good. But it can't always be accomplished, considering the fact that labor can last anywhere from fifteen minutes to fifty-five hours. In the latter case, a woman must permit herself to be relieved of some of her pain.

My chief objection to natural childbirth is that sometimes the choice of this method is prompted by fear. Some women have an irrational reaction to the idea of any anesthesia and believe that to lose consciousness is to surrender to a threatening unknown. Any woman with this dread owes it to herself to discuss it openly with her doctor early in her pregnancy. With his help, she may be able to dispel her fear. He undoubtedly will point out to her that most childbirth anesthesia is administered very moderately: a woman is given enough to lessen her pain but not enough to make her lose consciousness. He will probably assure her that he is aware that every mother wishes to be conscious for as long as is feasible, and that he wants her to be too, because it is better for her and for the baby. An excessive dose of anesthesia that knocks a woman out completely is potentially damaging to the baby and should never be used. Discreet use of medication—such as Demerol, which during labor relaxes a woman and blunts her pain—is often warranted and sometimes mandatory. Recent studies suggest that the baby, too, experiences some pain in the birth process. Medication given to the mother, threfore, also can ease the baby's discomfort.

If the circumstances are right and the woman's motivation is clear, natural childbirth can be a profound experience. The woman who goes through the preparations for natural childbirth usually receives very helpful prenatal education and comes into delivery emotionally prepared for the event. If she has a deep conviction that a baby will be the central experience in her life and that she wants to share the event fully with her husband, her baby, and her doctor, I understand her, admire her, and want to support her.

Perhaps one of the finest aspects of natural childbirth is the total involvement of the father. It took me a while to get used to the idea of having a young, anxious, and bewildered father looking over my shoulder as I dealt with the pressures of delivering an infant, but I've finally learned to accept his presence. I've also come to believe that in sharing the climaxing event of pregnancy a couple undergoes a baptism that can make them, as marriage part ners and as parents, stronger, closer, and more mature throughout the rest of their days.

XIII

The VD
Epidemic

Who gets VD?

The young. The poor. The lazy. Streetwalkers. (Not call girls: they are canny about self-care.) Homosexuals. People on drugs. People who are uninformed. And, above all, people who don't care, either about themselves or about anyone else.

All those people add up to quite a segment of our total population and constitute a virtual VD epidemic out of control.

Blocked by Ignorance and Indifference

The record of modern medicine in treating venereal disease in all of its forms is unassailable: VD is totally treatable. However, before a disease can be treated it must be detected and brought to the attention of a doctor. In our society, finding the people who have VD remains a major problem, particularly because the infection sometimes presents either no symptoms or symptoms so innocuous that they can be readily ignored. The people most vulnerable to the disease are either ignorant or indifferent, or both, and seem to remain unaware of the diligent although not very effective health-education efforts of the public authorities.

Partly because there still is—and perhaps always will be—a social stigma attached to venereal infection, far too many people remain reluctant to present themselves for treatment. The rather cynical attitude that gonorrhea is not much worse than a bad cold just isn't true. Gonorrhea has developed some stubborn new strains that require considerably more persistent treatment than does the average bad cold.

Are we deluding ourselves about eradicating VD? Yes, unless we take the one necessary rational step: we must develop better ways *to prevent* the disease. But we certainly can't achieve that prevention by high-minded denunciations of today's sexual practices. Prevention of VD will have to come from the same resources that wiped out smallpox, polio and other health threats: the research laboratories.

And we *must* prevent VD. Presently, to cite but a single example, public-health officials in California estimate that ten per cent of all persons between fifteen and twenty-four are afflicted and that some children as young as ten are suffering from syphilis and gonorrhea; in fact, 3,500 cases have been estimated for persons between ten and fourteen.

159

Based on these statistics, we had better give the problem some serious thought.

And the governors and state legislatures who speak of their "grave concern" and then look the other way had better give the problem some serious thought, as well. For instance, despite the alarming California statistics mentioned above, a November 1971 vote of that legislature failed to override Governor Reagan's veto of Assemblywoman March K. Fong's bill to make it easier for venereal disease instruction to be offered in the public schools.

Let's you and I take a hardheaded and realistic look at VD. First, we are talking not about one disease but about several, each of which is quite different. The two most common venereal diseases in this country are gonorrhea and syphilis. They differ entirely and are caused by totally unrelated organisms. They are also diagnosed through separate procedures. Additionally, they present dissimilar symptoms, if any, and the course of each, if untreated, is different. Yet they do have some traits in common. Both are caused by very delicate organisms that do not survive if they are exposed to the air. Both are transmitted only from membrane to membrane, which means, for all practical purposes, through sexual contact. And both can be successfully cured by antibiotics.

Does Gonorrhea Deserve Its Infamy?

Gonorrhea, the most widespread of the two, shows up primarily on the genital organs. It can be transmitted by mouth, and doctors are finding a good deal of it in the rectum. Many homosexuals are habitually promiscuous, and gonorrheal infections spread rapidly among them. The infection is diagnosed by a smear—that is, a microscopic study of the cells from the affected area.

A man is given warnings that he ought not ignore—a discharge from his penis and painful urination—but an infected woman may remain totally unaware of her ailment. A woman with gonorrhea usually has a vaginal discharge, but many female disorders, including minor ones, cause a vaginal discharge and, therefore, a woman often has a tendency to let this symptom go unnoticed and untreated. As a result, gonorrhea can then spread through her other reproductive organs. Other symptoms of this infection are fever and pelvic pain. Gonorrhea, even if it is untreated, usually does not affect other portions of the body. Its most serious consequence is to cause sterility.

People do not eventually rot away as the result of a gonorrhea infection, but the disease can be painful and disabling. Like any other infection, it should be treated promptly, particularly since the cure is available and inexpensive.

The Underground Disease

Syphilis, which can be diagnosed by blood studies, presents more clear-cut symptoms than gonorrhea, but these symptoms have an insidious trait: *they disappear whether or not the infected person is treated*. This fact makes it all too easy for a person who is generally lax about health practices to dismiss the infection until it starts to do seri-

161

ous damage. However, in all fairness to many of the people who fail to seek treatment, syphilis does not always signal its arrival with symptoms. About half of the persons who contract syphilis remain free of symptoms.

The first warning of this infection, which usually shows up about three weeks after a person's exposure, is a hard sore or chancre on the skin or membrane of the infected organ. Because it is painless, this sore is often neglected in this primary stage, which is also, unfortunately, a time when the disease is highly contagious. To make matters worse, a blood test *is not positive* immediately after a person's exposure; it usually takes three to six weeks for the infection to reveal itself in his blood stream.

Untreated syphilis reaches its second stage in six to twelve weeks after infection, at which time it is still highly contagious. During this stage the symptoms include a skin rash, fever, sores in the mouth, white patches on the skin, and small wartlike growths in the genital area. These symptoms, too, disappear whether or not the patient is treated.

In its third stage syphilis can do a great deal of "underground" damage. The person may have no symptoms, and unless he routinely has blood tests he may not even know that he's infected. But eventually the disease will take a grave toll: it will destroy the major blood vessels of the heart or cause deafness, blindness, paralysis, or mental illness. Almost every doctor has had the experience of treating an elderly patient, the very embodiment of propriety, whose entire body is riddled by an unsuspected syphilis.

VD and the Newborn

Does VD infect a newborn baby? The threat is not nearly so dire as it once was. There was a time when an infant, in passing through the birth canal, would contract gonorrhea from an infected mother. The bacteria would lodge in a vulnerable area, the moist membrane of the baby's eyes, and within a few days the newborn would be totally blind. It is now a legal requirement for all infants born in hospitals to be treated preventively, within an hour after delivery, by the application of either silver nitrate or penicillin, whether or not the mother is infected. As a result, except for the very small proportion of babies still delivered outside of hospitals, this problem has now been totally eliminated.

Though a fetus can contract syphilis from its mother in the final months of pregnancy, a woman receiving routine prenatal care has blood tests done regularly. If she shows any evidence of syphilis or any other venereal disease, both she and her unborn infant can be treated effectively with penicillin or other antibiotics. Among impoverished people, however, many mothers get no prenatal care at all, and since they often live in a physical and social environment in which syphilis is an ever-present risk, they, unfortunately, are vulnerable to producing syphilitic babies who are born either dead or damaged.

How About the Other VDs?

Some of the other, rarer forms of venereal infections have recently been magnified out of all proportion. Three of these—chancroid, lymphogranuloma venereum, and granuloma inguinale—are prevalent primarily in tropical and subtropical areas of the world and are not commonly seen in this country. Only occasional cases occur here, and these develop mostly among black residents of the southeastern states. Furthermore, contrary to what many have been led to believe, all three of these admittedly serious but far from widespread diseases can be successfully treated with sulfa drugs or other antibiotics and we are *not* in danger of being overwhelmed by these unusual forms of venereal infection.

The Wrong People Worry

Are people concerned about the spread of VD? Indeed they are. But those most concerned are often the least likely to be infected—for example, women who have never had any sexual experience but who are terrified by what they have read about VD. They may suspect the disease in a neighbor or the checker in the supermarket or the attendant at the gas station, and it takes considerable persuasion on the part of others, including doctors, to assure them that, whether or not their suspicions are accurate, they are not vulnerable to infection through a nonsexual exposure.

Many a patient calls me about symptoms that can reasonably be considered alarming but that, more often than not, are not symptoms of venereal infection. Many very common vaginal disorders, such as trichomonas and moniliasis, evidence themselves by a discharge that a lay person might misread as a symptom of gonorrhea. Sometimes, too, a patient has a lesion that she is convinced is

164

syphilitic but that proves to be a herpetic ulcer—that is, a cold sore transmitted through oral copulation.

The physician's chief concern about these misleading symptoms is that any one of them may frighten a person into *not seeking* an examination and laboratory diagnosis. Surely it is better to *know about and cure* a condition— any condition—than to gamble on its not becoming acute. Today it is standard practice in most public-health clinics to give antibiotics routinely to all patients with suspicious symptoms instead of waiting for the results of tests. The medications do no harm and often provide treatment to many patients with VD who would never keep a return appointment.

The Case of Jan: Postdated Betrayal

At one end of the patient spectrum I see fearful, even panic-stricken, women; at the other end I see those who are neglectful and irresponsible. But most of the women I see fall into a middle category and generally react to a diagnosis of VD with disbelief. Many of them ask, "How could this happen to me?" And many of them also blame their lovers.

Jan was a patient in the middle group. She and Herb, both in their late twenties, were staff members of the public-relations department of a recording company. They were both unmarried and thoroughly experienced sexually, and they had been lovers for three years.

Then Jan began to make a name for herself professionally and Herb resented the competition. After months of bickering, they decided to go their separate ways. Herb, whose ego was badly battered, sought solace in other women. Jan, much too busy forging ahead in her career, did not seek a replacement. Four months after their separation—four chaste months for Jan—they drifted back together again.

After their reunion, Jan came to my office with what proved to be gonorrhea, which she had contracted from Herb, an informed, sophisticated, mature man who didn't have the remotest idea that he was infected. Fortunately, she had come to see me at once. Treatment was immediately rendered to both, and their infections were cleared up, although Herb's treatment was more difficult because he had been infected longer.

The Paths to Prevention

If any drive to conquer VD is going to succeed, it must be preceded by a change in public attitudes. We must no longer consider the disease a scourge for sins committed. Unfortunately, because today's sexual promiscuity accounts for the present upsurge in VD, great numbers of people in this country—most of whom are old or righteous or powerful—believe that the disease is exactly what the "sinners" deserve.

As I have previously stated, effective prevention is a must. For syphilis, this will probably require a vaccine: in fact, experimental work is now being done in order to develop one. For gonorrhea, in my opinion the means for prevention are available now. Every neighborhood drugstore carries a number of bactericidal preparations that can destroy the fragile bacteria that cause gonorrhea. These preparations are sold as ointments and lotions for combating infections on the external surface of the body. To make these substances practical as antigonorrhea treatments, it is necessary merely to encapsulate them so that they will dissolve only at body temperature. Then such a medication, in the form of a suppository, could be inserted into the vagina before intercourse, and as it dissolved it would release a bactericide that would destroy any gonococcal germs encountered.

No major scientific break-through is necessary to create such a bactericide. I believe that, through tests, one could be developed from chemical substances that are already at hand. I believe that the pharmaceutical companies could manufacture such a suppository or some other combative product quite soon after a substance has been confirmed as a safe and effective destroyer of gonococci.

Will Progonasyl Prove to Be the VD "Magic Bullet"?

As these pages are being written, scarcely known to the public but with state and federal government acknowledgment, one pharmaceutical company is conducting a study in Nevada with a drug which thus far shows high promise as a VD preventative. With prostitutes playing the role of guinea pigs (prostitution is legal in Nevada under carefully controlled circumstances) an oily liquid substance known as Progonasyl has proved virtually foolproof during the first two months of the investigative period.

A few drops of Progonasyl, an organic iodine previously used for vaginal inflammation, treatment of nose or ear infections and presurgery preparation of membranes, are inserted into the vagina. Following a three-minute rest period, protection can be expected for the subsequent twenty-four hours.

During this study, conducted with the all-volunteer cooperation of the prostitutes in twenty of about forty legal brothels in Nevada, only two of the girls contracted gonorrhea, which may have resulted because of missing the required daily dosage.

Nevada State Health Officer Dr. John H. Carr found that many of the prostitutes involved will not now have intercourse without the daily dosage. "From the data we've collected thus far," said Dr. Carr, "we feel we can say that the drug is an effective preventative. There have been no dangerous side effects, although about ten percent of the girls have withdrawn because Progonasyl created some irritations."

While Amerex Laboratories, developers of Progonasyl, point out that it is still in an investigational stage, and while obviously this drug is somewhat removed from being VD's "magic bullet," it is heartening that government and private industry do recognize that something must be found to stem, and then obliterate—and in the future prevent—the ever-increasing menace of venereal disease.

Common-sense Measures

Until VD prevention is a reality I will continue to suggest to my patients that they rely on simple common-sense measures to *aid* them in warding off infection. Such measures should be considered mandatory if a woman's sexual partner is virtually a stranger or a casual, hastily encountered acquaintance.

With such a sexual partner a woman should insist that he wear a condom. My concern here is based entirely on the need for prevention of venereal disease. Even if the woman is on the pill and is not worried about getting pregnant, the man should use this precaution. In fact, the man should also be wary of infection and ought to consider the necessity of protecting himself. I also advise a woman to cleanse herself thoroughly, externally and internally, after a random sexual encounter. Soap and water don't kill many germs, but they do wash away quite a few. A woman should take a shower and scrub her pubic area with soap and water—which, incidentally, will help her to get rid of any possible crab lice. And, of course, she should douche.

If I seem to be destroying the magic of sex with these blunt instructions, let me assure you that there is nothing magical about the gift that a venereally infected man bestows upon you and that you, in turn, may pass on to others. In fact, the protective routine that I have just described is similar to the one in which every intelligent prostitute engages after coupling with a customer. Such a girl takes good care of herself because her livelihood is at stake, and under some conditions her routine is sensible for many a woman.

Does "Follow-up" Work?

The war against VD, as it is being waged today, is primarily the responsibility of the public-health authorities.

In some ways these agencies are doing a noteworthy job. For example, it is possible for anyone to get treated for VD at a public-health clinic *without charge*. I am convinced that if this were not possible the present problem of combating the spread of VD would be infinitely worse than it is.

The basic flaw of the public-health system is that it is committed to a follow-up policy that seems logical on paper but that, in the fashion of most bureaucratic processes, is not too workable in actual practice.

Understandably, public-health officials believe that treating an infected patient is not enough: they realize that they must track down the source of a patient's infection and extend treatment to that person, too. Accordingly, everyone treated at a public-health facility is asked to cooperate by providing the names of his or her recent sexual contacts. Similarly, every doctor is required by law to report all cases of VD to the public-health department and the patients involved are expected to cooperate so that their contacts can be identified, sought out and treated. This system sounds very orderly, but all too often it doesn't work. I'll use my patient Barbara to explain why.

The Case of Barbara: Victim of Mischief-Making

I received a call one day from San Francisco from the mother of a young woman whose first-born I had delivered. Barbara's mother was very guarded in her request that I check her daughter for syphilis and that, furthermore, I keep the request a secret from Barbara's husband.

Since the blood studies that I had done on Barbara prenatally had consistently been negative for syphilis, I was

170

nonplused. I am very fond of both Barbara and her husband, whom I've known ever since they've lived in Los Angeles, so I did a bit of sleuthing. The story that I came up with was chilling.

Barbara's uncle manages a rock group, which he had sent on tour. While performing in Florida, one of the musicians had developed syphilis, and when he had provided the names of his contacts he had included Barbara's. The Florida public-health authorities had notified those in San Francisco, and they had passed the word along to Barbara's parents. I learned long ago that nothing is impossible where the gonads are concerned, so I did not arbitrarily dismiss the story. But as I checked I found out that Barbara had not even seen the musician in a year, had never had sexual intercourse with him, and had been in the hospital, under my care, as an obstetric patient when the contact was supposed to have taken place. The story was pure mischief-making on the part of the man, but it could have meant disaster for Barbara's marriage.

How to Wipe Out VD

Barbara's case is not typical of the day-to-day activities of diligent and responsible public-health workers, and I am not using it as a basis for my assessment of the worth of the public-health program. The fact is simply that the program *does not work*. Moreover, its failure is inevitable considering the size of the task being attempted and the small number of modestly paid people doing it. By the time a public-health facility treats a patient, gets the names of his contacts, and then finds those people—if it ever does—the original infection usually has already been passed on to

171

several other partners. Thus an initially difficult task becomes still more difficult.

VD *can* be eradicated, but not by a small corps of civil servants. It can be eradicated effectively only under the leadership of medical scientists and with the aggressive support of the public. We must first eliminate the old-fashioned attitudes about VD. Then we must harness our technology to the production of foolproof preventives of the disease. Until we do these things we are being ostrich-like about VD infections and they will remain with us.

XIV

Marriage:
A Mating
of Strangers

The trouble with marriage is that it lasts so long.

A relationship that starts out as fortification against spending a lifetime alone all too often ends up as a lonely, worn-out, bitter and barren arrangement. Our society continues to make it difficult for couples to quit while they're still ahead.

In too many marriages the partners either are strangers when they start or grow so far apart that they become strangers as the marriage progresses.

Why the Best Foot Forward?

We are burdened with a series of misleading myths that all but destroy marriage from the beginning. When we start courting, each of us puts our best foot forward. Both the male and the female are on good behavior during the courtship. The girl displays herself to her best advantage and behaves beguilingly: she smiles, smiles, smiles. As a result, the man has only a remote idea of the character of the person he's courting. However, he is not any more candid with her. His pursuit routine is laden with courtesy, generosity, and considerate deference to her wishes.

Thus it is small wonder that there is a grim day of reckoning when the two find themselves bound together in a relationship that has been sanctified by a pronouncement that includes a "till-death-do-us-part" clause. Because it is only after the sanctification that the poor living habits, the quick tempers, and the differences in personal tastes and paces exhibit themselves and start to put stress on the union.

Many young people today are taking a far more realistic course by living together before marriage. I don't mean just that they are going to bed together; I mean that they are actually sharing a household. That way their relationship moves out of the mythology of dating into the day-to-day realities of getting up in the morning, sharing a hasty breakfast, and coping with both the dull and the bright spots of the average life. When such young people decide to get married—and, more often than not, they *do* get married—their decision is based a great deal more on reality than it is on fantasy.

Mission Accomplished

Another myth of marriage is the "live-happily-ever-after" expectation which is a fairy-tale promise that too many brides consider fact before the wedding cake is cut.

Relentlessly programmed from childhood to get a man, many a girl, once married, settles back with a sense of mission accomplished.

A girl reared in a home where traditional values prevailed has usually been indoctrinated with the idea that her life must be subordinated to her husband's. When she takes his name, she is also expected to adopt his aspirations and his living patterns. She is supposed to empty herself of her own goals, her capacities for achievement, and her strivings for self-identification. In short, she is expected to abdicate her true self.

Another kind of girl believes that with marriage, her ultimate goal, accomplished she is home free. She thinks that she will just relax and collect her daily allotment of the unending happiness that has always been promised to her.

Of course, all of us know that this is not how married life is, though almost all of us would like it to be that way. Just being a young bride or a young mother is not enough to make a successful marriage. Unless a woman continues to have a strong sense of herself as a person—a changing person—and unless she struggles with her own growth as well as with her husband's, she functions as only a passive partner in a relationship that is bound to deteriorate.

Must a Person Work at Marriage?

Many patients complain to me that they feel that their marriages have failed, but surprisingly sexual incompatibility is *not* their major complaint. In fact, many a woman admits resentfully that the only part of her marriage rela-

175

tionship that is any good is the part that takes place in the bedroom: while the man with whom she shares the bedroom is her lover, the one with whom she shares the living room and the kitchen is a stranger or, even worse, an enemy.

When I have the opportunity to talk to a husband and wife together they often agree, with a bitter sigh, that perhaps they haven't worked hard enough at their marriage. Now there's a statement that appalls me! Marriage is a demanding relationship. It doesn't thrive if the partners goof off. But I don't believe that it actually needs to be *worked at*. If it requires "hard" work to keep a marriage viable, then that marriage had better be re-examined. Assuming that a woman is going to work at anything at all during her courtship and marriage years, I'd suggest that she work at being herself and at realizing her own potential. I advise the same for the man as well.

It's Not the Only Way to Go

Marriage is no longer the only way to go. A woman does not have to get married because she is pregnant, because she wants children, or because she wants an active sex life. Today's woman may *choose* to get married—most women still do—but even so she is in a better position now to make a well-timed, unpressured, free choice than she ever was in the past.

Nonetheless, there are still a great many pressures, spoken and unspoken, that persistently push many a young woman into marriage. Such pressures come from her peers and parents or stem from either a personal in-

176

security that can be offset only by conformity to society's mold or a feeling that her worth will not have been invalidated until a man has claimed her in a public ceremony.

The Case of Sue Ann: She's Taking Her Time

Today many women are able to resist those pressures, and this is particularly true among my younger patients. One such girl is seventeen-year-old Sue Ann, the daughter of a wealthy father and a stunningly beautiful mother who also is from a highly successful family. Sue Ann is uncomfortable in her parents' lavish home, which she refers to as "the mausoleum," and is indifferent to their hopes that she will go on to college. Something about her parents' pattern of effortless success has turned Sue Ann against them and against marriage. She rarely sees them register close feelings for each other, and their lives seem to be based on an ostentatious display of possession, with each considering the other just one more splashy possession.

Sue Ann wants out. She is having an affair with a young insurance adjuster, and she has told me that the day she becomes eighteen she will move out of her parents' home and in with her boyfriend. She knows that there will be a parental explosion; in fact, I think that she is looking forward to the scene. Is there a marriage in her future? She couldn't care less. She feels that if the affair lasts for perhaps four or five years she may want to have a child, after which she might consider getting married. As she sees it, she will have plenty of exploring of herself to do and a lot of time for doing it, once she is free of parental judgment, before she can make up her mind about her future.

177

The Case of Dolly: No Stampede

Dolly, twenty-two, is living with twenty-seven-year-old Jim. Both have good jobs and neither has ever been married. Dolly is pregnant and delighted about it. There is nothing to keep them from getting married except the fact that Dolly isn't ready to take such a final step.

The past four years, since she left her parents' home, have been the happiest in Dolly's life. She has broken away from not only her parents but also their conventional values and the ominously religious overtones of her childhood. She has enjoyed her independence, enjoyed finding Jim and learning to love him, and enjoyed becoming pregnant by him. She is determined that neither of them will be stampeded into marriage. They may get married after the baby is born, but she will not let her pregnancy be the key factor in their decision.

The Case of Sharon: Marriage-Resistant

Sharon seems to me to be marriage-resistant, although I have never confronted her with that opinion. In her mid-twenties, Sharon is a successful career woman. She has been having a long and happy affair with Bill, a forty-two-year-old physician who is happily married but has a roving eye. At no time has Sharon badgered him to free himself of his marriage and marry her. Nor does she ask for any financial support. She recognizes that his profession makes many demands on his time and that he has family responsibilities. In fact, weeks often pass without their seeing each other.

As head buyer for a chain of department stores Sharon has a full life of her own, including a great deal of travel. She has a good income and many friends and has had many opportunities to marry. But none of these opportunities has seemed as attractive to her as her independence plus Bill. Sharon lives her life exactly the way she want to. She is competent, competitive, sought after, and successful in her roles as woman and executive, and she definitely does not want to add to her life the role of wife.

Getting Even

Most women have a better second marriage *if they end a first bad marriage soon enough.* The marriages that are truly corrosive and damaging are those that go on and on, long after all feelings have ebbed—love, sexual attraction, even interest—with nothing remaining but a muted and unadmitted drive to get even for the wasted years. ·

The reasons that people give for prolonging a marriage are rarely honest ones. They will tell you that they feel responsible for their spouses, that they can't bear to inflict pain, that they could never make it themselves. They will say that they owe it to each other and, above all, to their children to stay together. But I have yet to meet children or young adults who are, in any way, better off because a bitter, resentful marriage was extended for their sakes. Some of their parents' hatred has inevitably spilled over on them and their own chances for good marriages may well have been jeopardized.

The Case of Liz and Lou: Relentless Bickering

Liz and Lou placed their children above everything else throughout their marriage. They were both raised in middle-class Jewish homes where family solidarity was stressed. In the first five years of their marriage they had three children, all of whom were planned and happily anticipated. The trouble was that they had never openly talked about how they believed the children should be raised.

Liz diligently went to study groups and workshops and decided that she wanted to raise the children permissively. She assured Lou that being accepted by their peers was the most important experience the children could have. Lou, the son of a rabbi and a strict disciplinarian, was outraged by the liberty extended to the children and the way, according to his standards, they exploited that liberty.

As a result, the marriage progressed through twenty years of unrelieved bickering. The children, who watched their parents battle with each other over them, now have neither the security nor the self-respect that their parents planned for them. Furthermore, they have been told again and again how much they owe to their parents. Lou and Liz now admit that as soon as the youngest child leaves home they will separate. But I see little chance that either of them will reconstruct a new life. More likely they will both spend their time trying to collect the gratitude that they feel is due to them for the sacrifices they have made.

The Spouse as Monster

In many cases, the same pressures that impel two people to get married deter them from breaking up their marriage.

Personal insecurity is often a strong factor: each is afraid that he will never find another partner. The prospect of additional financial burdens also binds people together against their own impulses, particularly in states whose laws require a man to continue to be shackled with the economic responsibility of his ex-wife.

Society also places many obstacles in the paths of those seeking divorce. We tend to stigmatize as a failure a person whose marriage doesn't work out. Then when a couple decides to face up to that stigma and start divorce proceedings, one of them has to build up a case against the other. Thus the early happy years of a marriage are obliterated from memory and only the wrongs, the lapses and the injuries are remembered and documented, often vastly magnified.

How to Cope with Infidelity

Does infidelity tend to break up a marriage? Yes, it still does; but I believe that it shouldn't in this increasingly progressive world. Since a good marriage remains a good marriage despite many mistakes made by both partners, why should the mistake—or even the deliberate act—of sexual transgression be allowed to destroy an otherwise fine union?

If a woman tells me that she can't bear the humiliation of her husband's infidelity, I suggest that she ask herself why. What made him restless? What sent him wandering? I ask her to question herself not in an attempt to get her to accept the blame for the infidelity—because I don't think that infidelity is necessarily blameworthy—but because I have found that it is helpful to a woman to have this kind

181

of self-appraisal triggered. After looking at herself critically, a woman often comes to the conclusion that she has been coasting on past glories. If she then resolves to change, that resolution frequently saves what has been a good marriage. Variously, in an attempt to win back her husband, a woman taking a fresh look at herself sometimes discovers that she has outgrown her husband and has become qualified for a relationship with a new man.

Men seem to be much less capable than women of accepting marital infidelity, perhaps because men suffer more than women from sexual insecurity. What could be more revealing of sexual insecurity than the insistence that a bride come to her marriage bed a virgin? There are still many men who make this condition a requirement of marriage.

Is a Marriage Succeeding or Surviving?

Infidelity is not the major threat to marriage today. That threat is boredom, which results from the partners' growing apart without recognizing what's happening while still retaining debilitating dependence. Many marriages assaulted by boredom continue only from a force of habit. Most marriages do not really succeed; they survive. Marriage partners pay heavy prices for endlessly postponing the day when they will bring their grievances out in the open and break away: they drink or engulf themselves in work or refuse to let go of grown children.

The Case of Janet and Bob: Sex Was All

Janet and Bob followed a familiar pattern. When they met, in their late twenties, she was a waitress in a bar and he was a department-store executive.

They had both already had extensive sexual experience. They immediately clicked sexually and had a rapturous affair. But their relationship should have stopped when the rapture ebbed, because sex was all that bound them to each other. Instead, they married and had two children. By the time the children were in their early teens, Janet and Bob could no longer even feign interest in each other. Without common interests their days, and nights, began to drag endlessly.

Janet went back to work "to kill time," and both started drinking heavily. They rarely came home evenings, saw little of their children, and engaged in bitter strategies to escape each other. A friend of theirs persuaded them to talk with a marriage counselor, who advised them to separate for a year. They agreed to do so, but they never quite got around to acting on the recommendation. Instead, the hatred deepened, and one night Bob's frustration over his wasted life exploded. He beat his wife into unconsciousness. His two teen-agers had the harrowing experience of calling the police and seeing Bob taken to jail and Janet taken to the hospital.

Bob and Janet are separated now, and both are fighting what seems to be a losing battle with alcoholism. The children are on their own, having cut themselves off completely from their parents. Neither Bob nor Janet was irretrievably warped when they first met. A stagnant marriage simply brought out the worst in both of them.

Is Marriage Doomed?

I do not think that marriage as an institution is doomed.

183

It is natural for human beings to pair on a one-to-one basis. I have noticed that even in communes, where everything including child rearing is shared, sexual partners are *usually not* shared. But those commune pairings, if they are free of social pressures, tend to be rather short-term.

If we could enter into marriage without all-or-nothing expectations, the relationship would have a better chance. Some of the freedom that is characteristic of many affairs would infinitely strengthen most marriages. No one expects an affair to last forever. It lasts for as long as it's good. And while it lasts its participants have their independence, sense of worth, and the feeling that love, not a legal commitment, is binding them together. What marriage would not profit from these same endowments?

Young people are not destroying the institution of marriage; they may indeed be saving it. I have experienced few events more pro-marriage than the wedding ceremonies planned and carried out by some with-it young people. These youngsters write their own services and pledge only what they really want to commit themselves to. They wear their festive in-group clothes and play music that really speaks for them. The candor which such young people bring to marriage—and with which they perceive themselves and their expectations for the future—may prove to be the salvation of the institution.

Multiple Marriages

Although many marriages among youngsters fail, at least today they can walk way from a marriage with fewer backward glances than previous generations could. Divorce, to young people, is not necessarily a symbol of failure; it may mean a second chance. In my experience I have found that most people who remarry do much better with the second marriage than with the first. In such cases perhaps the first marriage should be thought of as in-service training for the one that follows. All marriages cannot be expected to last forever, but the solution for bad ones does not lie in banishing marriage as an institution. We should encourage the alternative of multiple marriages, not simultaneously, but successively. Many people could be enriched by endless self-discovery if society considered it normal rather than flighty to go through a series of four or five marriages in a lifetime.

Knowing Our Changing Selves

If the suggestion that people should keep changing seems to be a prescription for instability, so be it. Being stable should not be the ultimate goal in life. Each of us is potentially a changing, growing person, sometimes fickle, sometimes constant, sometimes able to give, sometimes needing to receive. It is this fluctuating self that each of us must guide through a series of relationships with others.

XV

The Super Orgasm:
Myth
or Reality?

There is no such thing as being good in bed—at least not all the time nor with every partner.

There is, in my opinion, a dangerous and dishonest sexual concept in this country. It is the concept of the orgasm as the ultimate experience. What is most conducive to experiencing sex *with* tears is the sense of failure many a woman has if she fails to have orgasmic climax during intercourse. Such a woman is convinced that she has failed as a woman and that, somehow, she has branded her sexual partner as a failure too.

What Not to Expect

Most men come to full climax every time. It's physiologically almost inevitable and not that much of an accomplishment. Many women reach climax with equal readiness, but there are some who rarely achieve it and some who never do. Any man who tells you that he can bring his mate to climax every time is probably lying. If not, his partner is faking: she is producing the responses that she thinks are called for in order to certify herself as a "sexual" woman and to validate her partner as a man.

For the most part, this frantic pursuit of the orgasm is fruitless. For most people, in most sexual encounters, the skies *do not* open up and lights *do not* flash blindingly. These fantasies have been concoted by romantic literature and pornographic magazines and films and, I regret to say, have been reinforced by self-styled professional sex experts. The pursuit of these fantasies helps us to lead young people—and many not-so-young people—to drugs, to group sex, and to sexual experimentation in terms of partners and positions in the hope that IT will happen or that IT will happen with more vivid excitement than ever before. But this quest is in vain. The sooner people return to realistic expectations concerning sex, the more fun and the more exciting sex will be. Furthermore, people will not feel so psychologically frustrated in their sexual experiences.

Now I am not downgrading either the orgasm, which is a satisfying physical and emotional sensation, or sex in general. Sex should be a source of pleasure and reassurance and joy *to both partners*, but it does not always transport them and they shouldn't expect it to.

Part of my professional responsibility is to help women to have sex without tears and to enjoy their experiences with men as fully as they can. Enjoyment, however, does

187

not necessarily mean *sexual climax*. A woman who has been fully aroused can often sustain a plateau of pleasure for as long as her mate can last, and such a woman, for whom this behavior is *a normal pattern of sexual response*, will feel completely fulfilled without an orgasm.

Let's Banish the Myths

In trying to reinterpret the sexual experience for my patients—many of whom have had extensive experience but are still bewildered about the basics—my starting point is that *people are all different*. That fact may seem self-evident, but it needs restating. Women come to my office feeling defeated because they are not reacting the way they believe they are *supposed* to.

Generally speaking, men normally have a higher state of sexual tension than women and, consequently, are more easily stimulated and satisfied. However, some very effective male sex partners frequently require a long build-up and some women closely approximate the usual male level of sexual readiness and require very little foreplay at all.

There is a common myth that a woman attains her height of sexual need at age thirty-five and at that point is an easy mark for any man who comes along. While that is true for some women, it is also true that some women of thirty-five have had all the sex they want—maybe a lot of good sex, maybe a lot of frustrating sex—and are all through.

One patient of mine in her early thirties was everyone's idea of the typical Hollywood bachelor girl. She had four lovers; mated with each of them once or twice a week; sometimes entertained two of them, in succession, on the same evening; and told me with some relish how great her life was. A year later, when she came in for a routine checkup, she seemed as pleased with herself as she had been before as she told me that she had had no sexual activity whatever for three months. She was no longer interested, and that fact didn't bother her at all. I think that her behavior was normal—*for her*—at both points in her development. She was also lucky to be wise and honest enough to accept herself as she had been and as she had become.

Another myth is that sexual pleasure continues undiminished throughout a lifetime and that sex is merely a matter of skill and stunts. This is not so. As we grow older we change, and one of those changes *in most cases* is a dwindling of sexual drive. Now this is not as depressing as it may sound. Some elderly people can maintain reciprocally pleasurable sexual activity; but some have sex only with great effort, making a gigantic production out of getting to the point where they can perform and doing everything the books tell them to, and many have willingly decided to forget it. I have had many a patient tell me that she feels foolish at her age trying to behave as if she were thirty or forty. Some women, in fact, say that it's a tremendous relief to them to be finished with sex.

Hurrah for the Difference!

Can people improve their lot, sexually speaking? Indeed they can. I can't provide a pat formula for them, but I can offer a number of suggestions ranging from surgery to true love.

Men and women come in different sizes and shapes. This

189

is true not only of their total physical beings but also of their individual components. The size of the male penis may vary quite markedly from one individual to another; the same is true of the female vagina. Additionally, both these organs also vary in placement: on some persons they are placed quite high in the pubic area and on others they are quite posterior, or close to the rectum. As a result, it is absurd to assume that any one specific way of joining these diversely placed organs will satisfy everyone. What stimulates one person sexually may discourage another. The key to satisfying any sexual exchange is in ascertaining what works best for the specific two persons involved in the union. If the most orthodox, face-to-face, man-on-top position is the most pleasurable, that's just fine: it doesn't mean that you're hopelessly square; it only means that the position is the one that is best for you. If, on the other hand, you and your mate find that a variety of sensory stimuli and a range of positions enhance your pleasure, that's fine too. Any two partners must experiment and test before they learn what suits them best.

Sexual experience also need not be limited to the genital organs. There is no body orifice or appendage that is "wrong" as an instrument for inducing sexual pleasure. Nor does the use of another part of your body in sex imply that your genital equipment is inadequate and that you therefore must resort to substitutes. Its use often means that you are inventive and imaginative and have discovered new ways of stimulating and satisfying your sex partner. My only word of warning is that you guard against using sexual virtuosity only for its own sake. Sex should

190

not just be a performance or a series of self-satisfying stunts. Remember that sex is a game at which two must play in harmony.

The Case of Lily: Who Was the Pervert?

Patients with sexual complaints sometimes present their problems to me either in shame or in anger. Lily exhibited both emotions. A twenty-four-year-old nurse from a conventional and rather strait-laced background, Lily had been married for three months when she came to see me. She had had some rather tentative premarital sexual experience with the man she married, but they had never established true sexual rapport. Lily's husband was a rather low-key person sexually, but he was unequivocally masculine. Lily was beginning to have doubts about him, however. She told me worriedly that there had been very little sexual activity between them in the three months of their marriage. That behavior wasn't normal, she felt, and finally she blurted out, "My husband's a pervert!"

As we talked I discovered that her husband, slow to be aroused, liked to indulge in pre-sex play with the lights on. Lily, however, believed that no one should gaze upon her naked body. Like her mother before her, she undressed in the bathroom, came into her bedroom in the dark, pulled the sheets up to her chin, and then got out of her nightgown to apprise her husband that she was ready.

That anyone trained as a nurse was still acting out this old-fashioned ritual astonished me. "You're quite right," I told Lily, "that there is a sexual pervert in your family, but it isn't your husband."

Then I told her what she subconsciously must have known: that her nonsensical behavior was depressing her husband sexually. Before she left my office she agreed to make an effort to change her pre-sexual ways. And good nurse that she is at following a doctor's orders, she did change, with the result that both she and her husband are enjoying sex—sometimes even with all the lights blazing.

The Case of Sonya: Why Not Talk about It?

Sonya came into my office in an open rage. She had been married for four years and simply wasn't going to put up with her situation any longer. She could not endure her husband. That is, she could not endure sexual relations with him because he chose to try to arouse her by blowing in her ear. While for many women this caress is exactly the magic touch necessary to arouse them sexually, for Sonya it was particularly loathsome. Moreover, since it was always a forerunner to sexual activity, she had also developed a loathing for sex.

Sonya had never told her husband of her feelings because she was convinced that a woman didn't talk about things like that. It scarcely took a doctor's training to suggest that she tell her husband that she didn't like what he was doing. Reluctantly she agreed to do so. Her husband, as would virtually any man, survived what certainly was not a soul-shattering rebuff, and their marriage is back on the track again.

One would think that because of the amount of information openly circulated about sex—how to do it, where to do it, and when to do it—cases like Sonya's would no longer be encountered. But I find that even a very informed and knowing person, who can talk glibly about sex in the abstract, often cannot discuss it openly with the one person who matters: the partner sharing the experience.

Many a woman cannot bring herself to express a sexual thought: a longing to try something different, the fact that a phrase habitually used by her partner in love-making irritates her, or the desire for her partner to give up his preoccupation with one part of her body and concentrate on caressing the part that would make her infinitely more excited.

Why shouldn't a woman talk about these things? It's *her* love life!

How a Doctor Can Help

Often the sexual complaints brought to my office are based not on psychological hang-ups but on explicit medical problems. Fortunately, I can do something about the latter. There is nothing that turns a woman off more completely sexually than pain or the anticipation of pain. Pelvic infections, structural abnormalities, and even ordinary wear and tear can create pain-producing conditions that cause women to dread sexual intercourse. A woman who is experiencing vaginal pain *cannot* respond pleasurably to sex: the intrusion of a penis is literally an assault and the friction caused by the movement of the penis in the inflamed or unlubricated vagina can indeed be agony.

Many women also experience vaginismus, a spasm of the vagina that makes the man's entry almost impossible. This spasm may be as unpredictable and as transient as spasm elsewhere in the body—in the lower back, for example— but if one occurs as a woman is preparing for sexual inter- course it may spell disaster. The spasm blocks the man's entry and if he tries to force his way in, the pain increases. The memory of such a pain can remain vivid, and thus the spasm may return at the next attempt at intercouse. By the time such a woman comes to see me, she is frequently convinced that she is all through sexually. The careful pelvic examination done on such a patient is performed primarily to convince her that she is not abnormal and that her vagina, which can receive my examining fingers and instruments, can easily accept her partner's penis.

Occasionally, however, in the course of such an exami- nation I do encounter a structural abnormality. Sometimes a thin wall of membrane, called a septum, covers a portion of the vaginal canal. This membrane may not be evident as the penis first enters, but it blocks the way before inser- tion is completed. Sometimes there are transverse bands of tissue across the vagina that make penetration almost impossible. Such abnormalities can be corrected readily by minor surgery.

Sometimes, in the hope that it will improve her sex life, a woman requests surgical correction of a too relaxed vagina. This is *not* an unreasonable request, since the delivery of a child sometimes stretches a vagina exces- sively. This correction also is a minor procedure.

Once in a while a woman of forty feels that she has suffered an over-all deterioration and, therefore, wishes to have surgical restoration. In such an instance I try to learn exactly why the request is being made. Sometimes such a woman may indeed be helped by surgical correction— although many women in their forties still have splendid, moist, firm vaginas—but other times her reason may be that her husband is sexually occupied with a twenty-year-old girl and she wants to resort to this last-stand measure in order to win him back. I would do surgery on such a woman only very reluctantly, because even the most successful operation in the annals of medicine would not give her the result she wants: to be twenty again.

The Case of Ella: A Therapeutic Triumph

My most gratifying experience with the above surgical procedure occurred accidentally, and I remember it vividly because it happened at the very outset of my professional career. I had been thoroughly trained to do post-partum repair and the important day finally arrived when I was to do a procedure by myself. Like most young doctors, I was somewhat overzealous. My handiwork left my patient, Ella, with such a small vaginal opening that I doubted that anyone would ever again be able to do a pelvic examination on her, let alone engage in sex with her. I was agonized by indecision. Should I tear down the surgery and do it over again or should I brave my way through it as it was? Since I knew that I would also do the post-partum checkup on Ella six weeks later, I decided to take my chances. I knew that, if necessary, I could always enlarge the opening.

During the checkup I did not advise Ella that I was barely able to introduce my fingers into her vagina in order to check the condition of her pelvis. Instead, I told her that I knew that I had caused her some discomfort and that she could expect some pain the first few times she again had sex with her husband. "Just think of it as another honeymoon," I said to her, mentally keeping my fingers crossed.

What I did not know—and did not find out until the next time I saw Ella—was that her husband had an unusually small penis. In the past, for the most part, Ella had been an absentee partner in sex, and finally, for the first time, she and her husband had experienced physical rapport and, thus, sexual rapport. Ella was the happy victim of my bungling!

The Female Circumcision

Another surgical procedure that I am often requested to perform on women who feel sexually denied is the female circumcision. In this operation the hood is removed from the clitoris in order to expose the sensitive gland, which is very responsive to stimulation. I do not advocate the female circumcision as a routine procedure, and I agree to do it only reluctantly. Usually a woman who requests it is suffering sexually not because of any structural abnormality but because of psychological hang-ups that are beyond the range of my expertise. Instead of taking the time to explore her inner conflicts, she seeks a short cut through surgery, convinced that once the operation is completed she'll be all set for the superorgasm that she has heard about so often. Such a woman is doomed to disappointment, and I would rather not be a party to that disappointment.

One female circumcision that I performed, however, was done for such a singular and—if you can believe it—such a sentimental reason that I recall the experience fondly. A seventy-eight-year-old woman, once renowned as a screen-writer, was married to a sixty-three-year-old man. They had always had an extraordinarily delightful sex life. When she came to me her husband had developed a cardiac prob-lem and she feared that he would overexert himself phy-sically to maintain their normal standards of mutual sexual satisfaction. She proposed to lighten his efforts by having a circumcision, and in her case her logic was entirely success-ful.

Flexing the Muscles

In most cases it is not necessary to resort to surgery to maintain pelvic health. A simple series of exercises, the Kegel system, which I have been advising almost routinely for the past fifteen years, is now enjoying popular accept-ance. It involves systematic contractions of the pubococ-cygeus muscle. Too many women are not even aware that they are endowed with muscles in the vaginal wall. In fact, we all tend to be unaware of any muscle that we do not consciously contract. Once a woman is taught how to sense the presence of that muscle—it must be done manually at first—and what it feels like to contract it, she can incorporate the exercise in her daily routine. I advise doing the exercise six times a day, with fifty contractions at each session. This daily total of 300 contractions, which can be done in a very few minutes, can make an enormous difference in pelvic health within three months. The activ-ity nourishes the area with an increased blood supply and provides a woman with strong muscles that are *subject to her control*. I don't think that this or any other system of exercises will convert an undersexed woman into a bedroom wonder, but it is a useful, positive, health-promoting means of maintaining vaginal tone.

An Abundance of Sex Organs

Most people solve their problems of sexual adjustment without help from doctors, or at least they try to. There are a great many things that two partners can do to help each other. First of all, they must realize that their genitals are *not* their only sex organs. All of the sensory organs are, in fact, sex organs. Soft lights and sweet music are not exciting only in the songwriter's imagination. These things provide authentic sensory support for a sexual build-up, which, generally speaking, is more important to the woman than the man.

Some women are aroused by what they hear—tender talk or suggestive talk or brutally frank sexual talk—and others are aroused by what they see. Although the nude female body is a powerful sexual stimulant for almost all men, the nude male body is not a similar stimulant for most women. However, many women are stimulated by today's fashions for men—such as tight, genital-revealing pants—and a lot of women also respond to the bodily rhythms of popular singers. Apparently women respond more to the implication of sexual prowess than to prowess itself. While we have always had Peeping Toms, we have rarely had Peeping Susies.

Touch is also generally recognized as a pervasive source

of sexual stimulation. The touch can be applied anywhere on the body, tenderly for those who prefer a stroking caress, punishingly for those with a taste for flagellation.

What is often forgotten is the importance of the sense of smell as a source of sexual stimulation. This sense seems to be enjoying a revival, but in this area the hucksters seem to be missing the mark. The campaigns against vaginal odor and vaginal taste advocate flower-scented feminine-hygiene deodorants and fruit-flavored douches. Many men, however, are aroused not by such delicate stimuli but by the strong scent of the normal vagina. In fact, quite a few women are excited by the pungent odors of male sweat and semen.

The Quest for Aphrodisiacs

The quest today is for a sexual stimulant beyond those available, an ultimate aphrodisiac that will produce the ultimate orgasm. Will such a chemical compound come into existence? Presently several chemical stimulants are effective under some circumstances for some people for specified—usually short—periods of time.

Testosterone, a male hormone, is being promoted for use by both men and women. If it does work at all, however, I think that its effectiveness is based more on the power of suggestion than on its measurable chemical action. The user seems to be perked up sexually by *knowing* that he has been given a dose of a mysterious, subtle substance of great potency. But it is exactly that potency that makes me reluctant to use testosterone or any other hormone indiscriminately. Furthermore, there are specific risks in prescribing testosterone. For one thing, if it is used for a prolonged period, it tends to masculinize women, causing hairiness, deepening of the voice, and other more subtle changes.

Alcohol, too, is advocated as a sexual facilitator, and in limited amounts it does lower inhibitions and induce relaxation, which is fine. But in unlimited amounts it blunts the sensory responses. A person may be having magnificent sex, but he is too foggy to know it. In fact, with one drink too many the male partner winds up impotent if not unconscious.

Drugs and Sex

Marijuana produces very much the same effect as alcohol. The moderate user is happy, relaxed, tranquilized, and often able to enjoy sex more than he would without a chemical assist.

Of all the psychedelic drugs, LSD probably does the most to expand all the sensations that are experienced under its influence, including the sexual ones. However, my patients who have used LSD admit that sex is only an unpredictable bonus. It may be either great or totally lost in other psychic preoccupations.

Young men who are particularly concerned with premature ejaculation are often rescued by the use of either amphetamines or "downers." With any of these drugs tension is lowered and the tactile sense is diminished and a man can continue to make love for what feels like forever. But what he does not appear to know—and what the sex partner of such a man will tell me—is that a man who is

heavily drugged is not a good sex partner despite an inter-
minable erection. As a person, he just isn't there, and a
woman might as well be in bed with a zombie.

One drug that seems to have a very specific effect as a
sexual stimulant is amyl nitrite. This drug is a vasodilator—
that is, it expands the blood vessels. Amyl nitrite is commonly used for patients suffering distressing symptoms of
cardiac disease, but sexual experiments have found that
sniffing the contents of an opened capsule immediately
before the sexual climax produces an exaggerated sensation. Indeed it does: the system receives an enormous
physiological boost when it is already functioning at a
peak. As a result, the system also experiences doubly stimulated heart action, which is medically unsafe.

But the search for new sexual experiences is not the
prime motivation of drug users. The really committed
users are little interested in sex. They are searching instead
for ways to shift psychic gears, and by the time they have
taken enough drugs—particularly hard drugs—to achieve
their desired mental states they are out of business sexually. And they don't care.

The Orgy Updated

Some people think that they will find a magical aphrodisiac in group sex. Group sex is not new; we used to call
it an orgy. What is new about group sex is that it is now
openly advertised, at least in the underground press;
soberly studied by social scientists; and indulged in by
otherwise conventional middle-class people. A number of
my patients have already talked to me about group sex.

201

Their first reports were glowing. Group sex is a great lark, they assured me. In addition, like newcomers to many experiences, they had missionary zeal and tried to entice others—sometimes including their doctors—to join their groups. As the months went by, however, their enthusiasm dwindled until, finally, they stopped talking about the activity and, quite probably, no longer indulged in it.

I know a few people who have stayed with a "swingers' group" for more than six months. Most have ultimately admitted that the essential experience of sex is really not magnified by being multiplied. Many have also told stories of failure. In the end, it seems that privacy is mandatory for the majority of people in their sexual relationships. Some men have found themselves totally impotent at orgies. Some women have admitted that, once the action started, they preferred to be spectators or faked their responses. Very few have experienced the explosive, incredible orgasm they sought.

Sex as a spectacle can quickly become a bore. Group sex becomes dull sex and watching the live sex staged in bars and "adult" theaters becomes tedious. As to the sexual displays in pornographic films and magazines, if you've seen one—or five or ten—you've seen them all. Sex, to be exhilarating, must have the elements of surprise and wonder; watching will never compare with doing.

I have come to the conclusion that there is no valid, universal aphrodisiac *except change*. That element is the newness that makes drugs and other stimulants *seem* effective. Variations in sexual partners as well as in methods of love-making are provocative. The excitement of change may doom monogamy as a way of life, but that change is what makes self-renewing sexual delight available to everyone.

An Act of Love

Inconstant though love may be, I am convinced that, in the long run, it is the most enduring basis for sexual pleasure. It is possible for everyone to have a number of loves in the course of a lifetime; sometimes these loves even occur simultaneously. By love I do not imply either monogamy or fidelity. Love is not a contract; it is a communion. Sex without love—sex to fill the void of loneliness or exploitative sex or self-aggrandizing sex—is unrewarding and rarely lasts. Sex is a trusting act and must carry with it expectations of fulfillment. It must promise not ringing bells and flashing lights but a future of shared pleasure. Seasoned lovers also know that there will be shared pain and shared comforting as well. The unmarried pregnant women I see who are devastated by their plight are those who did not love or whose love was not returned; those who *were* loved, no matter what their decisions about pregnancy, are able to handle their problem with a proud courage that surely comes from a sense of their own worth.

The message of courtship, of tenderness, of tantalization, and of romance, is not "How about some action?" but "I love you."

XVI

The Battle for Sexual Rights

The fight for genuine sexual freedom, for men and women alike, must be fought on many fronts, social, religious, cultural and political. The most telling battles must be fought and won on the political front to effect changes in the body of laws that restrict sexual rights. At this time, the laws most directly under attack are those regulating abortion. But, there are many other laws which will have to be revoked or revised to make them conform with changing social attitudes: laws affecting marriage and divorce, adoption and responsibility for child care, paternity and inheritance, the rights to property and the rights to privacy.

The thrust for political power for women is no newcomer to the scene; but, in today's climate of revolutionary change, it has emerged with great force and eloquence in the Women's Liberation Movement. "Women's Lib" has become an euphemism for the myriad of organizations fighting for some aspect of women's rights. Some seek legal changes, some changes in social customs and attitudes, some in economic rights and privileges—and some seem intent only on cutting men down to size.

Political power can be exerted on many levels, from the local PTA to the National Organization of Women (NOW). The PTA may be the most effective group in which to fight for sex education in schools; NOW, perhaps the most vocal and militant of Women's Lib groups, might be the best vehicle to tackle long range national issues which require a change in our social consciousness before political action can be initiated. I, personally am particularly interested in the goals of Planned Parenthood, a responsible and highly effective organization which has pioneered in contraceptive research and education and has led the fight for legalized abortion. Also, I am on the side of the League of Women Voters in its continuing campaign to inculcate the women of this country with a sense of their political power and to educate them on current issues.

The Male-Dominated Judiciary

Actual achievement of Women's Lib goals will not be easily attained. As just one example of the fight the women's groups have before them let's look at the American judiciary and its handling of sex discrimination cases, which points up the difficulties in winning equal rights for women. A study, completed in late 1971 by Professor John D. Johnson and Charles L. Knapp of New York University Law School, examined court opinions handed down since 1870 and concluded that decisions pertaining to sexual rights ranged from "poor to abominable."

This indictment of the male-dominated judiciary goes on to say "judges over the years, with some notable exceptions, have failed to bring to sex discrimination cases those judicial virtues of detachment, reflection and critical analysis which have served them so well in other sensitive social issues."

A Supreme Court decision in 1873 was cited by Johnston and Knapp as establishing a female-discrimination attitude which for 100 years has influenced the law and lawmakers. Upholding an Illinois ruling that barred a woman from practicing at the bar only because she was a female, Supreme Court Justice Joseph P. Bradley wrote:

"The paramount destiny and mission of women are to fulfil the noble and benign offices of wife and mother. This is the law of the creator . . . It is within the province of the legislature to ordain what offices, position and callings shall be filled and discharged by men, and shall receive the benefit of those energies and responsibilities . . . which are presumed to predominate in the sterner sex."

Other prejudices the courts have demonstrated throughout the past century include discrimination against women in the areas of employment, access to public accomodations, jury duty, public education and criminal sentencing. The courts, say Johnston and Knapp, cling to the belief "that women are—and ought to be—confined to the social roles of homemaker, wife and mother, and gainfully

206

employed if at all only in endeavors which comport with their assumed subservient, child-oriented and decorative characteristics."

In the light of the above, the Women's Lib cry for "Woman Power!" takes on new meaning!

The Media and the Revolution

It's surprising what can be accomplished by the individual in today's climate of awakening awareness and instant communication. Germaine Greer, a self-pronounced non-joiner, has reached millions of people through her book, *The Female Eunuch*, aided by every arm of the media. I find Miss Greer to be a very engaging prophetess, perhaps because her militancy is not chauvinistic. In this connection, I must confess that many of the views expressed by some of the more militant Women's Lib leaders seem to be as biased and intolerant as the attitudes they are opposing. But, although I may bridle personally, I realize that political warfare is joined on the battleground of the media and that controversy and militancy serve to flush the enemy out of his defensive positions. Being male, it is emotionally difficult for me to accept many of the positions taken by spokesmen for the movement; and, being a gynecologist makes it impossible for me to ignore the physical and anthropological differences between man and woman. But all revolutionary movements need extremists to man the frontlines, and in the McLuhan era, the frontlines are the headlines. For that reason, I respect what Kate Millet and Betty Friedan have accomplished in helping make the revolution a reality. There is a qualitative difference between commitment and concern and it takes the total commitment of the Millets and the Friedans to win acceptance of a new, revolutionary philosophy.

The depth of the struggle for women's rights as fought by the more militant Women's Libbers can be seen in the variety of issues which are being argued by them. For example, one of the issues raised by NOW is the matter of semantics. The organization is seeking to eliminate the use of "man" in the English language as a suffix to denote a person, either male or female. NOW recommends that the word "one" being sexless, be substituted for "man" or "woman." Instead of salesman or saleswoman, we would say "salesone." This is the kind of an issue which I think serves a purpose. It's an interesting conversation piece and illustrates the psycho-social issues which permeate the movement. And it gets attention in the media, which is all to the good. But I think I should be excused if I want to devote my efforts to issues which I believe are more pressing and immediate, the issues to which I have addressed myself in this book. And I am confident that my attitude reflects that of many men who want to help the cause, but have difficulty finding a place in the ranks.

The word "media" has cropped up constantly as I tried to express my thoughts on the sexual revolution. Of the media, it's paradoxical that one of the prime targets of Women's Lib has been a most important influence in the liberalization of the public's attitude towards sex. I am referring to *Playboy* magazine and, as I write this, I have suddenly realized, that in some ways, I identify with Hugh Hefner. Both of us make our living from women's bodies, both of us believe strongly in women's sexual and political rights, but there is where the identification ends. I identify with women far beyond their physical beauty. In any event, the influence of periodicals like *Playboy* will play a most important role in woman's fight for sexual equality, a fight that cannot be won without winning to its cause a large segment of the male population.

Sex and the Single Grandmother

A fellow doctor whom I have long admired, the syndicated columnist Dr. Walter Alvarez, brought to my attention the story of Harlette Surovelle, a remarkable testament of what one person can accomplish, and a sixteen-year-old, at that!

Harlette was a senior at John Browne High School in Queens, New York, and a member of the High School Women's Coalition which was formed to unite girls from high schools all over New York City into an action group. Harlette was called before the National Commission on Population Growth and the American Future to testify on methods of educating teen-agers about contraception. She had come to the attention of the Commission because of her one-girl campaign in the New York City school systems.

Harlette's interest in the subject began when her hygiene teacher wrote on the blackboard all the methods of contraception she knew. One of the students then asked her which method she recommended for teen-agers, and she answered, *"Sleeping with your grandmother."* The reply struck Harlette as inadequate, to say the least. And her reaction was underscored some ten months after the lecture when one of the girls in her class had a baby. So

209

Harlette took the matter in her own hands and bought some birth control handbooks to distribute to fellow students. When she was advised that it was illegal for her to give them out, Harlette appealed to the Board of Education for permission to start a program in all high schools in New York City to provide birth control and VD information as well as referrals to physicians and other helpful information to students willing to attend the program.

One of Harlette's innovations was a "rap room" where the girls could discuss sex problems with an informed person their own age. Harlette learned that many of the girls didn't have the most rudimentary knowledge of the sexual or birth processes, many didn't even have a clear idea where babies came from. "I found," says Harlette as quoted in Dr. Alvarez' column, "that many of those girls who were sexually active were using withdrawal as a method of contraception and almost as many were using nothing at all." Harlette also found that some were taking their mother's or sister's contraceptive pills without knowing how they were to be used. Some took a pill just before they had sex; others, immediately after. And, of course, the pill is useless under these circumstances.

Harlette also tackled the problem of venereal disease which has reached epidemic proportions in New York schools. The VD program had featured an "educational" film which was so old-fashioned that it had lost all relevancy. Harlette pointed out that while kids were purchasing heroin in the back of the room, the teacher was showing a film about teen-agers smoking marijuana at a hippie party: and, then, when the subject switched to venereal disease, they were shown a film made in 1956

210

about a teen-age boy who takes a "loose woman" to a motel room, contracts venereal disease and then infects the nice girl next door who wanted to please him because he had taken her to an exclusive country club dance. Not very meaningful to the average student in a New York school!

It is difficult to evaluate the results of Harlette's efforts. But of one thing we can be sure, the young people who have availed themselves of the information dispensed by Harlette have a much more realistic knowledge of the problems and their solutions than those who have been exposed only to the classroom curriculum.

Harlette, in addition to the support of the High School Women' Coalition, is now receiving official recognition nationally. One girl, with conviction and initiative, can indeed work miracles!

Men's Lib, Too!

I don't want to imply from the emphasis on the role of women in the political struggle that men should not be equally responsible for taking leadership roles. As a matter of fact, it seems to me that implicit in the Women's Lib movement is liberation for men. There are many men who envy women with their freedom from the responsibility of family support, the hours together with the children while they are growing up, the opportunity to return to school after the children have matured, and the freedom to start a new career which will be rewarding personally, if not financially.

If Women's Lib achieves all its goals and women take an equal position with men socially and economically, all of us, regardless of sex, should benefit. In particular, men have a responsibility to liberate women in the area of sexual rights. "It takes two to tango" is an old refrain, but where the sex act is concerned it bears repeating. Too often the male has walked away from the dance floor when the music has stopped, leaving his partner to thread her way through the crowd alone. Women should no longer be forced to bear the burden of problems arising from the sexual act without support from society as a whole and the least society can do is to give her the full and complete right to make her own decisions regarding the protection of her emotional and physical health and her destiny as woman and mother.

I am not advocating the formation of a Men's Lib movement. Hopefully, men will not take the Women's Lib movement as an attack on their male egos, but will analyze the goals of the various women's organizations and support them in every way possible when they serve the purpose of freeing women from the cultural chains which have bound her for so long. In the end, support of these goals will win freedom for the men, too.

XVII

Questions
and Answers

The times have indeed changed for women and their doctors. Some of the changes have been drastic, as we have seen in these pages—and we may well wonder what the future holds in store and how soon more changes will occur.

One thing is certain: today's woman has gained almost all the equality with men that, until recently, she was too timid to demand for herself. She has gained this equality chiefly through her insistence for sexual freedom. As a consequence of shedding the sexual shackles for all time, she has been able to force men to accept her in a new light and to see her as a new and different person.

Nevertheless, there are still some questions that we should consider. What do the changes of the past fifteen years add up to? Are women really better off now than they were then? Have their lives been improved? Are they happier and healthier? What victories—and what defeats—have they experienced in the sexual revolution?

Here are some of the questions that my patients ask me and that I frequently ask myself:

How has the climate of sexual permissiveness affected women?

For the first time, the idea that sex should be enjoyed by women as well as men is being openly discussed and acted upon. Traditionally, we have always learned from our elders, but today we are learning from young people. Young women are candidly enjoying sex, and their older sisters—and even their mothers—have decided to follow their example. As a result of this new attitude, women in general are more willing to experiment with variations in sexual intercourse. The departure from the face-to-face position in intercourse is certainly not an innovation exclusive to today's young generation. The innovation is that the refinements and varied pleasures of sexual contact, once considered the privilege of only the leisure class, have become the common practices of everyone.

Has opposition to abortion as an accepted procedure dwindled?

There has really been very little decline in official opposition to abortion among most religious and political leaders. There continue to be organizations, including medical groups, that make the anti-abortion position their cause. Furthermore, all the weight of our tradition of

214

righteousness and morality—by which I mean a sense of sexual shame—supports those who resist change.

At the individual, private level, however, the prevailing opinion is quite different. Women welcome the increased availability of abortion realistically, sensibly and with considerable relief, and most doctors whose experience with unwanted pregnancy is similar to mine feel as I do.

In fact, in a recent federal survey forty-nine per cent of the adults questioned favored permitting abortion when parents have all the children they want. Reflecting the current public concern about overpopulation, the results of the survey indicated a dramatic change in public attitudes.

The nationwide survey, conducted by Opinion Research Corporation for the Commission on Population Growth and the American Future, involved 1,700 white and black men and women from sixteen years of age up. The majority also believed that the government should help to provide abortions for those in need and should make birth-control information available to anyone who wants it.

Are married women more open-minded about extramarital experiences now than in the past?

Yes, they are definitely more open-minded about such experiences, and they also look upon them with considerably less guilt.

By letting down the barriers to pornography, have we promoted promiscuity?

No. In fact, I think that those events have occurred just

215

the other way around. The generally permissive sexual climate has cleared the path for the explicit movies and books. While it still may be a shock to see so many young people on dates buying tickets for X-rated films, I don't think that viewing such films results in sending to bed together couples who were not already sexually intimate with each other.

How do parents feel about the sexual revolution?

My experience is primarily with mothers, who, I feel, mostly tolerate the changes but do not welcome them. The typical mother of a teen-age girl will talk with me rationally about the advisability of informing young women about contraception, but when I move the conversation to the personal level and suggest that we do something precautionary for her daughter she tends to bristle. Invariably such a mother welcomes the solution of an abortion for her daughter if an unwanted pregnancy does occur.

Are there new developments in medical science that help a woman in her quest for sex without tears?

Changes and improvements in devices for contraception and new techniques for performing abortions are evolving constantly. In addition, two recently developed medical specialities have the potential for resolving many serious problems. One of these, fetology, the science of the development of the fetus from the moment of conception, has already produced a number of methods of early detection of congenital defects. The other, genetic counseling, offers prospective parents a realistic forecast of the heredity outlook for their unborn children.

216

Has the sexual revolution created new problems for the doctor?

Yes. It is infinitely more difficult to practice medicine today than it was when I started. A doctor must know much more, because there are many more options for him to offer his patients and he must exercise much keener judgment in making professional decision. In addition, patients are far more knowledgeable today than in years gone by and they challenge their doctors constantly. They are inquisitive and critical, and sometimes even hostile. They ask many questions: Why? Are you sure? What will happen if I don't? Why did it go wrong? Some of this pin-pointed questioning arises from commendable curiosity, but some of it is in understandable retaliation against the medical profession's centuries of self-ordained mystery and smugness.

Do patients understand sex better than they used to?

There certainly is a greater quest for more understanding of sex, but the truth is that there is still very little real knowledge. Even doctors and psychiatrists don't fully understand sex. Despite how most sex manuals define sexual knowledge, there is more to understanding sex than knowing the anatomy of the penis and the vagina. What makes the man-woman thing tick—when and why and with whom—remains an unknown quantity.

Has the sexual revolution created more problems than it has solved?

No, but it has created quite a few. Let me cite some of those that continually come to my attention:

217

- An increase in VD, with very little increase in the understanding of it and almost no change in the attitudes toward it.
- Unrealistic expectations concerning sex. Not every woman is going to be transported to ecstasy by every sexual experience despite all the current propaganda to that effect. The manifestations of frustration and self-doubt and the sense of failure remain constant.
- Almost no illegitimate babies available for adoption by barren families.
- The need for society to take initiatives in helping to rear both the children of single mothers and the children of married parents who have abrogated their responsibilities, because the next generation is, to one degree or another, everybody's responsibility.
- A widening of the already large generation gap. Many parents are secretly envious of the freedom that their youngsters enjoy, and this envy is expressed in disapproval, rejection, martyrdom, imposition of guilt upon the young, and ultimate alienation.

Is today's woman relinquishing anything precious in exchange for her freedom?

Yes. Today's woman is relinquishing her former total dependence on the man to make the important decisions in her life. Increasingly, however, she is seeing her traditional right to male support as demeaning rather than precious. She can now look forward to making her own choices of her role in life and her sexual partners.

Today's woman tends to be honest and realistic. She is not problem-free, but she is better equipped than ever

218

before to recognize her problems and she now has the freedom to try to solve them by herself.

The sexual revolution has shattered the role of a woman as a possession and has offered her the uniquely human opportunity to become a self-realized individual.

Is it safe to stay on the pill indefinitely?

We do not know for sure how long it is safe to take the pill, but many have taken it for more than ten years. Studies would indicate that it is safe to take the pill for at least ten years. Beyond this, medical knowledge in the contraceptive field is increasing every day, and I am sure that the current pill will be replaced by an even better contraceptive soon.

How many abortions can a person have?

There is no limit to the number of abortions that one may have. However, there is a small risk to future fertility and to life with each abortion. So naturally the more times one has an abortion, the greater the risk. An abortion done properly and with no post-operative infection does not harm the uterus.

Can a woman conceive while breast feeding?

Yes. However, a woman's fertility is markedly reduced during nursing.

Does the contraceptive pill increase or decrease the sex drive in the young female?

It has been my experience that women both single and married who use the contraceptive pill have an increased

219

sexual drive as compared with those women using other contraceptive methods. I have no explanation for this except possibly the woman feels more free sexually because she has full confidence in the contraceptive ability of the pill and the fear of pregnancy is eliminated.

Does excessive sexual activity in young life result in an early end to the sexual drive?

No, quite the contrary. The more sexual a person is in youth the more sexual he will probably be in old age and the longer he will be sexual.

Is there a greater risk of infection from oral-genital contact than in sexual intercourse?

Probably not. Syphilis can be transmitted orally, as it can with fingers or any other appendage. However, the syphilis organism is very sensitive and easily killed and is spread less easily by oral-genital contact than through sexual intercourse. Gonorrhea, the most common venereal disease, is rarely transmitted by oral-genital contact. There are multitudes of other nonspecific and nonserious infections that are possible; however, the mucous membranes of the genitals as well as the oral areas are usually resistant to these organisms.

I am married and have been on the pill for several years but plan to have children when we are in an economic position to raise a family. I am concerned about reports of cancer developing in the daughters of mothers who have taken estrogen. What do you advise?

220

Back in the early 1950's a synthetic hormone was given to women to prevent miscarriage. This estrogen, Stilbestrol, is chemically totally different from any of the present-day contraceptive pills, as well as the estrogen found in the body normally.

Recently, the New York State Department of Health found five cases of cancer of the female organs in twenty-year-old girls, whose mothers had taken Stilbestrol while carrying their daughters. This finding is a bit alarming, since this kind of cancer rarely occurs in young women. Although these five cases do not provide proof that Stilbestrol caused their cancer, it is enough evidence to warrant further observation. And since the drug is probably not effective at preventing miscarriage, we should stop giving it to pregnant women. However, I see no cause for alarm for those women who are using the pill.

Postscript

While I was writing this book, I often had the feeling that events were moving faster than my typewriter, that the book would be outdated before it was published. From my standpoint, I wish it were so; that progress in the field of sexual rights would snowball, making books such as this unnecessary.

Unfortunately, the forces of reaction are more stubborn and resourceful than I have given them credit for. At this writing, just prior to publication, the governor of my state has vetoed a bill permitting unmarried minor girls to receive contraceptive help from doctors without parental consent, giving as his reason the belief that such a bill would serve to break down the family unit by removing the parent's authority (as if an unwanted pregnancy is constructive to family unity!); and a judge in New York has set precedent by appointing a legal guardian for an unborn child to prevent its abortion. These actions by the executive of one state and the judiciary in another (states in which the legislators have led the way in liberalizing the state laws), indicate the difficulties and duration of the struggle for sexual rights.

But governors can be defeated at the polls and judges can be reversed. Final victory will go to those who have right on their side; right backed by knowledge, social action and political pressure.

I hope that in some small way this book will help in that struggle.

ABOUT THE AUTHOR

Dr. Boyd Cooper practices in Los Angeles, California, specializing in gynecology and obstetrics.

When he was serving his residency, Dr. Cooper was assigned to the Florence Crittenden Home for Unwed Mothers where he provided parental care and performed deliveries. It was while on this service that he became familiar with the complex emotional, social and legal problems of these young women and active in the movement for the reform of abortion laws.

Dr. Cooper is a pioneer in the research and use of the contraceptive pill and conducted research projects on the pill for Eli Lilly & Company and Syntex Products. He is currently engaged in chromosomal research.

Dr. Cooper lives in Sherman Oaks, California, with his wife and three children.